Praise for

THE AGE FIX

"This is a wonderful read for anyone trying to look and feel their best. The best part of Dr. Youn's many tips is that they will not only improve your outward appearance without surgery, they can also help improve your overall health. And, as all doctors know, a healthy glow starts with a healthy life."

—Dr. Travis Stork, ER physician, host of the Emmy Award–winning, syndicated series *The Doctors*, and bestselling author

"Dr. Youn is a frequent guest on my show, and I can say without a doubt that he's a cut above the rest!" —Rachael Ray, TV host and *New York Times* bestselling author

"A refreshingly honest look at what *really* helps you turn back the clock. This definitive guide is a must-read for anyone who wants to look younger and sexier, using real food and natural techniques as your medicine, without spending a ton of money."

—Haylie Pomroy, #1 *New York Times* bestselling author of
The Fast Metabolism Diet and *Fast Metabolism Foods Rx*

"Dr. Youn is an innovator in the field of plastic surgery. This easy-to-read book informs, inspires, and entertains. I highly recommend it!"

—Robert Rey, MD, MPP, star of *Dr. 90210* on E!

"Dr. Youn succeeds in putting forth all you need to know about skin from the inside out; even if you can't be one of his actual patients, you will *feel* and *look* like you are after reading it!"

—Dr. Jennifer Ashton, senior medical contributor,
Good Morning America; co-host of *The Doctors*

The
AGE FIX

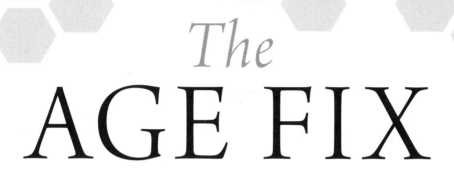

A Leading Plastic Surgeon Reveals How
to Really Look 10 Years Younger

ANTHONY YOUN, MD

with EVE ADAMSON

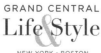

GRAND CENTRAL
Life & Style
NEW YORK • BOSTON

Copyright © 2016 by Anthony Youn, MD
Bonus chapter copyright © 2017 by Anthony Youn, MD
Cover design by Claire Brown and Connor Cowden; cover photograph by Image Source/Getty

Illustrations by Matthew Cushman

Grand Central Life & Style
Hachette Book Group
1290 Avenue of the Americas
New York, NY 10104

www.GrandCentralLifeandStyle.com

Originally published as a hardcover edition in 2016
First trade paperback edition: December 2017

Grand Central Life & Style is an imprint of Grand Central Publishing.
The Grand Central Life & Style name and logo are trademarks of Hachette Book Group, Inc.

The Hachette Speakers Bureau provides a wide range of authors for speaking events. To find out more, go to www.HachetteSpeakersBureau.com or call (866) 376-6591.

The publisher is not responsible for websites (or their content) that are not owned by the publisher.

Library of Congress Cataloging-in-Publication Data

Youn, Anthony.
  The age fix : a leading plastic surgeon reveals how to really look 10 years younger / Anthony Youn, MD, FACSW with Eve Adamson.
    pages cm
  Includes bibliographical references and index.
  ISBN 978-1-4555-3332-9 (hardback)—ISBN 978-1-4789-6066-9 (audio download)—
ISBN 978-1-4555-3331-2 (ebook)—ISBN 978-1-4555-3330-5 (trade paperback edition)
  1. Aging—Nutritional aspects.   2. Aging—Prevention.   3. Skin—Health and hygiene.
  4. Beauty, Personal.   I. Title.
  RA776.75.Y67 2015
  613.2—dc23
                                                                              2015028985

Printed in the United States of America

LSC-C

10 9 8 7 6 5 4 3 2 1

This book is lovingly dedicated to my mom,
who never seems to age.

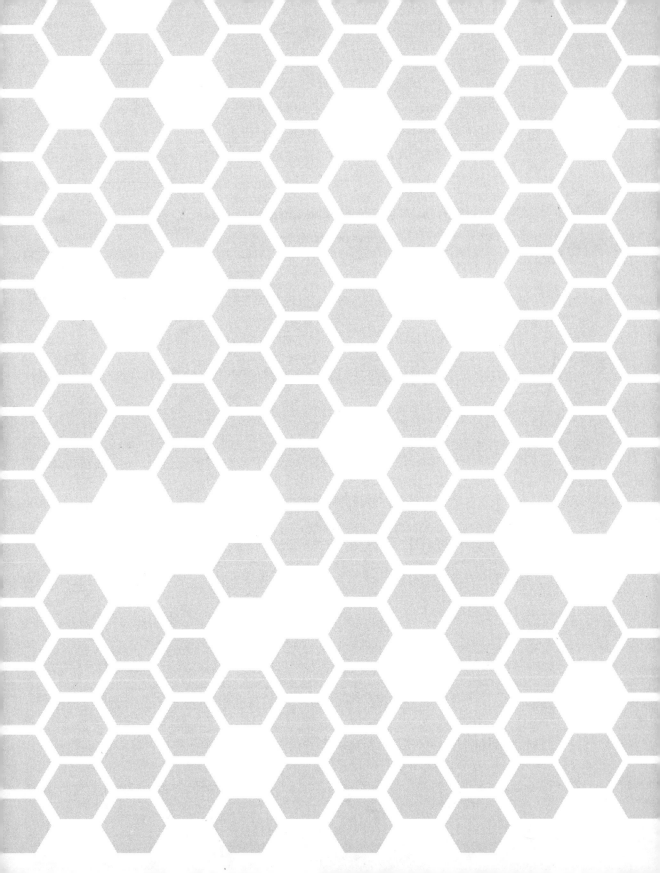

Contents

INTRODUCTION

As a preteen, I had a feature that interfered with my confidence. I had a genetic condition called mandibular prognathism, sometimes called Hapsburg jaw. This condition causes the lower jaw to grow much faster and larger than the upper jaw. The result: My jaw began to grow, and grow, and grow, to my horror and consternation. There I was in junior high school, and my jaw and I (I thought of it almost as its own entity) made Jay Leno look weak chinned. Believe me, when you are a skinny, geeky eleven-year-old Asian kid with Coke-bottle glasses and a bowl haircut who is already terrified to talk to girls, a monster chin does not help the situation at all.

At first, my chin was merely prominent. Then it became an architectural feature. When you could set a drink on it, I wanted to hide in my room. High school is humiliating enough, but for a nerd with a monster jaw, it's pretty much unbearable. Every day, my chin grew larger. I examined it in the mirror. I used a hand mirror to check my profile. Yep, there it was, in all its glory, preceding me into every room I entered, practically announcing my presence: "Hey, everybody! Look at me! I'm Tony's ginormous chin! Oh, and Tony's here, too. He's back behind me somewhere."

I wanted to do something about it. I wanted plastic surgery, but my parents didn't like the idea. They thought I looked fine. (Of course they did. Sheesh!) However, by the time I finished high school, even my parents couldn't deny that my chin had taken on a life and a personality of its own. They finally consented to plastic surgery, and after that, everything changed for me. The young man I was becoming on the inside finally resembled how I looked on the outside. That was exactly what I was going for—I didn't want to change my face out of vanity. I just wanted to look like myself. What that surgery did for my self-esteem (and eventual recognition by members of the opposite sex) inspired me to become a plastic surgeon.

But this isn't a book about plastic surgery. This is a book about bringing your outside in line with your inside. This is a book about options. Maybe you are fifty, and although you hear fifty is the new thirty, what you see in the mirror is only a distant relation to how you remember yourself in your thirties. It doesn't have to be that way. Maybe you are forty but you still feel twenty-five, and your reflection startles and alarms you because it isn't the you that you feel like inside. I have answers. Maybe you are thirty and you are seeing the first signs of aging, like crow's-feet and forehead wrinkles, but you still want to rock a bikini. You can.

Sure, aging is natural, but does it have to happen so soon? I can't stop you from aging, but I can stop you from looking like you are aging. Aging happens more rapidly and dramatically in some people than in others, but there are remedies, solutions, and fixes that don't involve surgery. In fact, most of them shouldn't involve surgery, in my opinion. I may be writing myself out of patients, but I can't recommend that everybody go under the knife. It's simply not necessary. You can look younger, your skin can look smoother and brighter, and you can feel better without plastic surgery. This book will show you how.

Nonsurgical techniques can't solve every problem, and I'll be sure to level with you when that's the case, but with the advent of technology and chemistry behind the antiaging revolution, they sure can solve a lot of problems that you may have right now. And I'm going to tell you all about those nonsurgical techniques—I'll also tell you when those so-called miracle products don't really do much of anything and when you should save your money for something more effective or enjoyable (like a glass of wine or a massage—both have antiaging properties!).

Fortunately for all of us who are concerned with the superficial effects of aging, there are many, many effective products—from topical creams to fancy technological devices—that really do make a difference. I strongly believe that nonsurgical treatments are the future of plastic surgery, and a source of real and meaningful solutions for those of you out there who would do almost anything to get rid of the sagging neck, the fine lines, the sun damage, the cellulite, or the bags under your eyes—anything except surgery.

In this book, I'll address all your cosmetic issues and show you everything you can do to turn back the clock and correct the minor (and even some of the major) things that really bug you, from stretch marks to wrinkles, from natural frowns to varicose veins, from yellow teeth to body odor. For each problem, you'll get a full range of strategies, from natural remedies to the latest cutting-edge products and tools. I've even provided you with an Age-Fix diet plan, to keep you younger from the inside out, starting today.

I'm not that guy on an infomercial trying to sell you a miracle. I'm the guy you can go out for a drink with after work and know he'll tell you what's what. Wouldn't it be great if you had a friend who happened to be a plastic surgeon, and you could ask that friend anything and get a straight answer? That's me, and that's this book.

I'll also be perfectly frank with you about what you can expect with different levels of treatment. And despite the premise of this book, I'll even tell you when plastic surgery really is the only good option. (This is true sometimes, but less often than you might think.)

In other words, this is a book you can trust, with information you can use, that really will make a difference in the reflection you see in the mirror. It is a bible of cosmetic remedies. Pick your trouble spots and watch the calendar flip backward. Watch your skin tighten, your flab firm up, your wrinkles melt, and your eccentricities morph into assets. All of this is possible... *without surgery.* The answers lie within these pages, so let's get an age fix. Let's dive in. You're going to come out looking like a younger version of you.

1 | YOUTH and BEAUTY

How beautiful do you feel? How young do you look? These are questions that plague my patients, sometimes more than they need to, but as a plastic surgeon, I tend to be the one people come to for the answers to their questions about how to look more beautiful and, especially, younger. They come to me looking for an age fix.

They've come to the right place. In order to give my patients the solutions they want, I've spent the past sixteen years researching the secrets of plastic surgeons, dermatologists, makeup artists, and dieticians, and I have compiled all the solutions I've discovered to nearly every beauty problem right here in this book.

But that doesn't address the real question I want you to think about as you read through these chapters. I want you to think about what beauty and youth really mean to you. Are they important? Are they too important? And do you seek them out of fear, or do you seek them out of an impulse to love and take care of yourself?

When I think of beauty, the first thing I think of is my wife. She is beautiful to me, and always will be, no matter what her age. I also think about my mom. Although she is nearly seventy, her skin is flawless, with barely a wrinkle. Yes, I may have injected a little Botox (just a little!), but she's never had any actual surgery. The real reason she looks so young and beautiful is because she eats the right foods and lives the right lifestyle, and especially because she takes care of her skin. Every time she visits me, she goes on a shopping spree in my office. This petite Korean woman brings a trash bag with her and empties my cabinets into it. This lotion, that moisturizer, that antioxidant. She loves trying new products and takes at least two of each for the road. And she uses all of it. It really shows.

But how can someone who doesn't have a plastic surgeon in the family continue to look younger and better, just like my mom has done? My mom has already given you some clues. You don't have to spend an awful lot of money, undergo painful procedures, or burn your skin with lasers. You begin with a firm foundation: a healthy life. You eat well, you move, and you enjoy yourself. And if you can use a few products, devices, and home remedies to tweak your results? All the better.

This book will be your guide. It is a collection of information about how to address every possible beauty and cosmetic issue—an antiaging resource providing information on a wide range of appearance-improving strategies from natural to chemical, simple to super-high-tech, short-term to long-term, including a dietary intervention for maintaining vitality and youthfulness. From face to feet, you'll get the inside scoop on how to bring out your youngest, freshest, most glowing self. The solutions I offer are actually fairly simple, whether you are looking to treat that small perceived imperfection that drives you crazy or do a complete makeover on your face and other parts of your body.

But I also want to emphasize that I'm not here to tell you what I think is wrong with your skin or your shape or the relative size or firmness of any part of you. I'm not here to judge how young or old you look, or to weigh in on any of the eccentricities, irregularities, and signature features that make you who you are. We all have our beauty issues, and as we age, we take on more . . . battle scars, stretch marks, crow's-feet, and laugh lines are all badges of honor, the beautiful patina of a fully lived life. There is nothing wrong with having any feature if it doesn't bother you.

But what if it does bother you? What if it interferes with your peace of mind, your happiness, your self-esteem (whether it should or not)? Knowing I'm a plastic surgeon, is there something you would like to tell me or show me, maybe in confidence, that you wish you could fix? Something that you wish was different—younger, smoother, smaller, larger, tighter, or higher than it is right now? Maybe there is *just this one little thing* that keeps you from feeling good about yourself—an eccentricity or an irregularity or an age-related alteration that you don't like when you see it in the mirror. If that sounds like you, then I'm here to help. No judgment, just solutions.

FROM DIY TO OTC TO OR

In this book, I cover many different types of techniques, gadgets, products, and remedies, and even a few procedures that can maximize your assets and help you look younger. Some of them you can make at home. Some of them you can buy at your local pharmacy. Some of them require a prescription from a medical doctor. Some (just a few) require an operating room. I offer you many options because I want you to have a lot of choices.

Maybe mixing up a face cream in your own kitchen sounds like your idea of fun. Go for it! I've got recipes. Maybe spending a little extra money on a really high-quality wrinkle cream or eye cream is in your budget and on your list. Great! I'll tell you where to spend your money and where not to waste it. Maybe you are Botox curious. Cool! I'll tell you what you need to know (and allay your worst fears). Maybe having your doctor use a high-tech laser on your stretch marks or sagging skin is totally you. Awesome! I'll tell you exactly what you should know before you go.

From nose to toes, I've got secrets that will rejuvenate you, but before we get into those chapters, I want to take just a short time to explain the differences between the kinds of treatments I'll be talking about.

Several levels of intervention are possible for just about every body part you would like to improve. Essentially they come down to these four:

1. **Natural:** These interventions use the products of nature, like fruits or milk or oil, many of which you probably have in your own kitchen. Can you say "DIY"?

2. **Chemical:** These interventions use chemistry to your benefit. Many of these chemicals are derived from or synthesized from natural compounds but have been altered to be stronger and more potent. Some of these products are available over the counter, and some require a prescription from your plastic surgeon, dermatologist, or other doctor.

3. **Technical:** These are the gadgets, devices, and machines that aren't surgical in nature but that can make a real difference in how your skin looks. They includes things like lasers, pulsed light, ultrasound, and radiofrequency waves. These devices are very expensive, so most of the time you would require a visit to the doctor to use them. There are a few less powerful gadgets that you could invest in for home use.

4. **Surgical:** These are (obviously) the interventions that require a surgeon's practiced hand and include things like brow lifts, facelifts, breast augmentation, and liposuction. This is not the focus of this book, which is about the many, many nonsurgical antiaging resources available to you. However, if you do decide that you need plastic surgery for an issue that can't be handled any other way (and these do exist—I'll be sure to let you know), I'll give you a little bit of information to guide you.

Some people definitely gravitate toward the natural side of things. They like mixing up their own skin-care remedies at home and saving money on a DIY approach. Others are more likely to try more intense treatments because they want faster or more dramatic results. Some people enjoy the process of finding the most effective chemical treatments, like over-the-counter creams with the latest age-reversing ingredients. Some people like the fun of technical gadgets that can make them look younger. A few people may opt for a surgical procedure. You will have your opinions, but I will give you all the best options. Generally, I recommend chemical and technical solutions as the most effective, but I like many natural treatments, too. I'll give you the information you need. Let's talk about each one of these so you can best choose, in any of the following chapters, which kind of intervention will be best for what you want to do.

Natural

Natural methods are the least invasive. Unfortunately, they tend to be the least effective. However, there are some notable exceptions, which I will mention in this book—natural treatments that really do make a noticeable difference. This is good news, because a lot of people are very interested in natural treatments. I receive inquiries all the time from people seeking suggestions for less expensive, easier alternatives to the skin-care products and treatments that we sell in our office and that I've shared on TV. Many of these inquiries come from people for whom paying $20 for an over-the-counter retinol cream would be a stretch.

I once received a handwritten letter from an older woman who complained about terrible sun spots. She lived on a fixed income in rural Ohio and was hoping that I had a solution for her. She wrote, "I'd love to buy the ZO stuff you've talked about on TV, but to afford it I'd have to cancel my weekly Bunco night at Cracker Barrel with the ladies!" I wrote her back and told her to try one of the recipes you'll read about in chapter 4. It costs only pennies per application and, given enough time and dedication, can create some really nice changes. Four months later, I received a thank-you card with "before" and "after" photos of her. She looked great! Although some of her sun spots were still there, she had a definite improvement and was very happy. She recommended my sun-spot treatment to all her Bunco friends. So if you see a bunch of sun-spot-free faces at a Cracker Barrel Bunco party in rural Ohio, you'll know exactly what they're putting on their skin.

Making your own skin-care products at home is just one way to use natural treatments. Occasionally you can buy products with natural ingredients, but to me, natural remedies also include lifestyle shifts, like eating natural foods to look younger and practicing stress-management techniques to relax worry lines. I provide many recipes for homemade products throughout this book, and I share only those that I believe actually make a difference—but not every remedy works for every person (and that doesn't just apply to natural remedies). However, if you are oriented toward natural products, then you will want to look out for these.

There are some definite advantages to natural treatments. For one thing, you will avoid exposing your skin to too many of the negative aspects of commercially available products, like potentially harmful additives, including dyes, fragrances, preservatives, or other chemicals that could cause an allergic reaction. Natural products also tend to be much less expensive than commercially available options. The problem with many natural options you might hear about out in the world (and especially on the Internet) is that they don't really do anything. For example, there are some ingredients from your own kitchen that really do make a difference, like yogurt, but others that don't, and still others that may actually cause an allergic reaction just as distinct as one you might get from a commercially available product.

Unfortunately, there isn't an all-natural (or even a nonsurgical) solution to every cosmetic problem, but when they work, they can be a nice and inexpensive option.

Chemical

Chemical treatments include things like chemical peels, prescription treatments, and commercially available skin-care products. Although nonsurgical and generally noninvasive, in many cases they can dramatically reverse aging. I once had a patient, Candace, who came in to see me for a facelift. She was in her late fifties and complained about wrinkles and fine lines on her face. She also didn't like the subtly loosening skin on her neck, her age spots, and her sun damage. I thought Candace was an appropriate candidate for facelift surgery, so we made plans to perform the operation six months later, at the time of her preplanned vacation. She asked me if, in the meantime, there was something she could do to improve her skin prior to surgery.

I started her on a combination of tretinoin, 4% hydroquinone, and alpha-hydroxy acid creams, at a total cost of less than $200. Three months later, Candace called to cancel her surgery. She was so happy with how much better the combination of creams made her skin look that she felt she no longer needed the facelift. She saved over $8,000, didn't miss a day of work, skipped going under the knife, and, best of all, looked great.

The advantage of chemical treatments over natural treatments is that they tend to make a more dramatic difference in less time. Natural products are gentle and slow, and chemical treatments can be too harsh for some people, but when they work, they tend to work pretty well. I recommend many chemical treatments throughout the next few chapters that I like and believe to be quite effective.

Of course, chemical treatments don't always work for everyone, usually because people may react poorly to them. Some chemical treatments may be too harsh, causing irritation, rashes, itching, or peeling. In some cases you might be able to find a less intense version of the same treatment. After seeing the great results that Candace achieved with my cocktail of skin creams, I decided to recommend that same combination to my mother. If it worked for Candace, who had terribly damaged skin, how great could it make my mom's skin, which was nicer than the skin of 95 percent of women her age? Not nice at all! She reacted horribly to it, she developed a rash, and her skin flaked off all over. She looked like she'd forgotten her sunblock and fallen asleep while sunning herself on a beach in Mexico. As many people can attest, hell hath no fury like a Korean mother whose face looks like the inside of a pomegranate! I started her on soothing moisturizers and steroid creams, and she wore a surgical mask over her face in an attempt to hide the shame. Within two weeks, her skin finally cleared up, thank God! (My dad and I were also extremely thankful!)

Technical

Technical intervention is fun for those of us who like gadgets. These treatments can be divided into two groups: at-home and in-office. These days, consumers have access to all sorts of at-home gadgets that promise results similar to those we get with the treatments we perform in our offices. These devices range from the tried and proven (such as at-home microdermabrasion) to the large, bulky, and sometimes unrealistic (an at-home version of our in-office cellulite treatments). Then there is the advanced technology (like home laser hair removal) and devices that are just plain ridiculous (like a device that supposedly causes your nose to change shape). While none of these gadgets can typically approach the results of surgery or in-office treatments, some of them can be a valid alternative for people who want to save money and address issues in the comfort of their own homes.

In-office cosmetic treatments are now a multibillion-dollar industry. What started back in the 1990s with simple but effective CO_2 ablative laser resurfacing has expanded over the last several decades to include laser hair removal, wrinkle reduction, skin tightening, tattoo removal, acne reduction, and even what I call the Holy Grail of Plastic Surgery: noninvasive fat reduction. Yes, you can now lose fat and inches without having to diet or exercise! It's amazing how far in-office technology has come. In fact, according to the American Society of Plastic Surgeons, over the last dozen years the number of nonsurgical cosmetic procedures performed in the United States has increased

144 percent, while the number of cosmetic surgeries has actually declined 12 percent! Today, it's all about getting results without going under the knife.

Unfortunately, sometimes the hype of these technological devices precedes proof that they actually work. In fact, some device manufacturers use what is essentially a flaw in the approval system to allow them to sell and even market devices that are declared safe, but not necessarily effective. Cosmetic medical devices can be considered "FDA-cleared" or "FDA-approved." A device can be considered FDA-cleared if the manufacturer and the FDA agree that it is very similar to another device already on the market and is deemed safe to use. Becoming FDA-approved is a more rigorous process, used for devices for which there aren't other, similar approved models on the market. What makes it even more confusing is that some devices may be FDA-cleared for one indication but used and marketed by physicians for a completely different indication. For example, some devices may be FDA-cleared for pain reduction, yet plastic surgeons use them to reduce fat.

So the big question is: Which devices actually work? Plastic surgeons and dermatologists have an inside joke regarding obsolete devices or ones that never worked in the first place:

PLASTIC SURGEON #1: *So, Dr. Shmo, I'm thinking of buying the Super Laser. How is it working for you?*

PLASTIC SURGEON #2: *It's working great! As a very expensive coat hanger.*

Many older plastic surgeons have several of these types of devices sitting in their offices gathering dust. I once had a plastic surgeon who worked in my building move out to a different office. On his way out, he dropped off a skin-rejuvenation machine that he had bought about eight years earlier for approximately $60,000. The device claimed to tighten the skin by deep-heating it, and was even heavily promoted on TV talk shows. He told me that he couldn't figure out how to get good results with it and ended up bequeathing it to me as a gift. "Maybe you can figure out how to get people happy with this," he said. Well, I'm not one for using old technology on my patients, especially technology that was never proven to actually, consistently work, so it sat in my storage room for months. I finally decided to put it on eBay and sold it for $4,500 to a laser-refurbishing company. I used the money to make a down payment on a fence to keep the scary dogs next door out of my yard.

In the upcoming chapters I will give you tips and advice on which devices work, which ones don't, and which ones on which the jury is still out. I hope I can keep you from wasting money and get you on the right track to using technology to remove the years. Because you may need that money for a fence.

Surgical

None of my patients actually want surgery, and I don't want to perform surgery on them. Surgery always has risks, and unless there is absolutely no other option available, I would prefer to do something less invasive. Sometimes this is the case.

A couple of years ago, a man came in for a consultation. He wanted to smooth his nasolabial folds. These are the lines that extend from the sides of your nose to the corners of your mouth, and they are typically shaped like commas. He was very flustered and said he had tried everything to get rid of them. He even went to one of those chain facelift centers (you know, the ones with half-hour infomercials on Saturday morning cable TV) and asked them for suggestions on how to treat his nasolabial folds. The "patient consultant" convinced him that their special lunchtime facelift would do the trick. She even pulled his cheeks back to show him how his comma signs would go away. After he'd paid $6,000 and undergone a painful two-hour operation, his nasolabial folds were still there. But now he had god-awful permanent scars around his ears to show for it. When he complained about it, the medical assistant told him that the doctor was no longer available to see him and that there was nothing else they could do. That was when he came to see me.

After $550 and one syringe of Juvederm, his nasolabial folds were gone. That was all he needed in the first place. Any plastic surgeon worth a nickel knows that facelifts don't treat nasolabial folds. Injectable fillers do. He emptied his bank account, underwent painful surgery by inexperienced hands, and gained permanent scars for nothing.

In other words, there are many, many times when surgery is not the answer. Most of the time, there are valid and even highly effective noninvasive solutions. The only major exceptions, which I will explain later in this book, are for breast augmentation, excessive hanging stomach skin, and drooping upper eyelids. In these cases, surgery is the only really good option if you find you can't live with your issue. Otherwise, you should never need to go under the plastic surgeon's knife, at least for antiaging issues. There are so many other fantastic and effective treatments you can explore that surgery can simply be a nonissue.

Doing Nothing

Finally, I'd like to give you one more option that you may not have fully considered. It might sound strange for me to give you this advice as a plastic surgeon and the author of this book, but here's a fact: As you age, you don't have to do anything.

Nothing at all.

Sometimes you are better off living with a cosmetic issue than trying to fix it. Sometimes you are better off letting aging take its course. Aging comes with its own sort of beauty, and if you don't mind an issue all that much, or if you are even proud of the badges of honor that mark your life experience, then don't worry about every wrinkle, every line, every crooked or uneven part. These are what make you *you*, and I would never tell you that you should fix them.

But if something really bothers you? If you know you could look and especially feel better, more confident, and more like yourself if you fix a particular issue? Then by all means, let's fix it!

2 | MYTHS ABOUT BEAUTY, SKIN CARE, and PLASTIC SURGERY

I've got a lot to tell you about what works, but before we dive into the truth and start remaking you so you look and feel younger than you do right now, let's get some of the untruths out of the way. People have some pretty funny and strange ideas about beauty, aging, skin care, and especially plastic surgery. I hear myths described as sacred truth all the time. Patients do it, parents and friends of patients do it, and even doctors themselves have been known to propagate a few beauty and plastic surgery falsehoods.

As a plastic surgeon, I would like to clear up some of this misinformation because it gets in the way of the truth and the things that can provide real results and make a real difference in how young you look. Let's start by separating beauty truth from beauty fiction. Here are some of the most popular questions I get in my clinic:

Q. *Is it true that all celebrities get plastic surgery?*
Not all, but a lot of them do. Quite a lot, in fact. And if you have been operating under the false impression that people who naturally look better than the rest of us are the ones who get to be celebrities, you may be surprised at how many of them resort to the knife. There is a huge amount of pressure in Hollywood to stay looking as young as possible for as long as possible. To many celebrities, plastic surgery is a sort of business expense.

However, plastic surgery doesn't always go well for celebrities. Just like anyone else, celebrities sometimes pay too much for bad results. When you think of celebrity plastic surgery, you might think of some who've had obvious bad work. Or maybe you are inspired by those celebs who've admitted to having plastic surgery and look great after. Celebrities like Sharon Osbourne, Julie Chen, and Kris Jenner come to mind. However, you should know that for every celebrity plastic surgery you know about, there are dozens—no, more like hundreds—of celebrities who've had plastic surgery that is so good, almost no one can tell it's been done. No one but a person with a trained eye, that is—like maybe a plastic surgeon.

For example, I suspect (although I have not treated them and cannot say for sure) that the following celebs may have had the following surgeries:

* Julia Roberts—nose job? (To my eye, her nasal tip looks thinned, as if cartilage was removed from it.)

* Helen Mirren—facelift? (It's very unlikely that someone her age has a neckline so sharp and youthful without surgery.)

* Julie Bowen—breast implants? (Although the change is modest, her chest now appears to me to match her frame more perfectly than it did before.)

The reason why I mention them is that these are three of the most beautiful celebs in Hollywood. We like to think that their beauty is effortless. But it's not. Like us, celebrities have pimples, wrinkles, sun damage, droopy breasts, and cellulite. Unfortunately, unlike most of us, they also have teams dedicated to making them look good. They have stylists, hairdressers, facialists, plastic surgeons, dermatologists, aestheticians, personal trainers, dieticians, masseuses, and more. So how can you, a regular person, compete with this? You don't need to be a millionaire and have a team of experts to look and feel young. All you need are a few dollars and the suggestions in this book to rock the red carpet as well as (and in some cases, even more beautifully than) the Hollywood stars.

Q: *Do only excessively vain people get plastic surgery? Am I being shallow to care about looking younger than I really am?*

You're not vain or shallow to want to look younger than you currently do. I tell my patients that each one of us sits somewhere along a continuum or a scale indicating how much we are willing to do to look younger or better than we do right now. For some people, all they are willing to do to improve their appearance is to eat better and use creams on their skin. Others may be willing to undergo treatments at home, such as at-home microdermabrasion and handheld laser treatments. Some people are willing to have in-office lasers and other noninvasive procedures, whereas others may consider injections of Botox and fillers. A small percentage of people are willing to go under the knife to enhance their appearance. Still others truly don't care about altering their appearance at all, and just let nature take its course. I suspect, however, that the latter category doesn't include any of you. If it did, you probably wouldn't be reading this book!

But no matter where you fall on this spectrum, whether you stop at creams or go all the way to surgery, no one should judge you for caring about your appearance. We have such a multitude of noninvasive, minimally invasive, and surgical options to look younger today that it's a shame if you don't take advantage of whichever of those you feel comfortable with. My patients include all types of people, like accountants, homemakers, pastors, teachers, doctors, social workers, nurses, engineers, police officers, firefighters, and—my favorite—military personnel. Vain? Shallow? I don't think so!

Q: *I'm not sure about surgery. Can I just do facial muscle workouts to keep my face from sagging?*

Maybe you've seen the programs for facial exercises to keep your face young, tight, and uplifted. Can you really do the equivalent of push-ups and sit-ups for your face? If exercise tones your abs or lifting weights at the gym tightens up your deltoids and biceps, shouldn't this approach work for your facial muscles, too? You certainly can strengthen your facial muscles if you feel like it, and stronger facial muscles might help you hold that big smile for photographs longer, but the bad news is that this will not combat sagging.

Unfortunately, your face and your abdomen don't sag for the same reasons. The abdomen can sag when you lose muscle tone, but faces sag due to a loss of collagen and elastin in the skin. It's true that the platysma muscle of the neck can become stretched and droopy with age, but no amount of exercise has ever been shown to cause this muscle to lift and tighten.

Once on the *Rachael Ray* show, I tested a facial exercising device. Not only did it not work, but everybody laughed at the person using it. Double humiliation! Don't waste your money on these, and don't waste your time making weird faces and repetitive movements in the name of a tighter, younger face. It's not going to help, and you're going to look mighty silly.

In fact, repetitive facial muscle movements combined with a loss of collagen and elastin can actually cause more wrinkles. It's the same concept that's behind smile lines and crow's-feet and forehead wrinkles. The more often you make a certain facial movement that creases your skin, the more likely that crease is going to settle in and make a permanent home on your face. I once heard a rumor that Elvis Presley forbade his then wife Priscilla from lifting her eyebrows and crinkling her forehead, since he was concerned that doing this would cause her forehead to permanently wrinkle. While this story may or may not be true, the fact is, flexing the muscles of your face can worsen your wrinkling.

You've probably heard of Botox, the treatment that temporarily weakens muscles. (I'll talk more about Botox later in this book.) The reason Botox works so well is that it stops you from moving your face, and that's the best way to postpone wrinkles. There are some topical ingredients, like GABA and DMAE, which can temporarily tighten skin and theoretically smooth the muscle contractions that create wrinkles. Technically, these really shouldn't work, but some of them do seem to show results. There are even better things on the horizon, which I'll tell you about a little bit later in this book.

Q. *Can pillow wrinkles become permanent?*

If you periodically wake up after a hard night's sleep with pillow wrinkles on your face, you might wonder whether they're going to stick around. Your mother may have told you that frowning or looking cross-eyed too often could make your face "stick that way." What can I say—sometimes mothers are correct! Actually, sleeping on your face *can* cause wrinkles. A crease on any given day won't have an effect, but if you always sleep on your face or on your side, creasing your face in the same way night after night, the deep creases that are temporary in the beginning can become permanent over the years. These are called sleep wrinkles, and they are different from wrinkles formed by muscles (called expression lines). The best way to avoid sleep wrinkles is to sleep on your back.

I recognize not everyone can do this. Some of my patients say they can't sleep on their backs because it is uncomfortable, or they have breathing or snoring issues, but your sleep position is usually nothing more than a habit. Unless you have a medical problem like sleep apnea, or you are pregnant, it's worth a try. Do it for your face. Sleeping on your back is real beauty sleep, because gravity works with you, not against you. Here are some tips for better back sleeping:

* Put a pillow under your knees to make you more comfortable. This can also take pressure off your lower back.

* If you get congested at night, add an extra pillow so you can be just slightly propped up as you sleep. You could also try a breathing strip to help open your nasal passages.

* Consider a more supportive mattress. Memory foam can make back sleeping more comfortable, because it molds to your body and holds you in place.

* Try a cervical neck pillow. These pillows are designed to cradle your neck while you sleep and help prevent the dreaded neck spasm that many of us occasionally wake up with.

Beauty Secret

If you must sleep on your side, a satin or silk pillowcase will not crease your skin as much as a cotton or polyester pillowcase. If you insist on continuing to sleep on your face (old habits die hard … emphasis on *old*), I recommend 100 percent silk pillowcases. This will cause the least possible long-term damage in the stomach-sleeping position.

Or better yet, check out the **Juverest pillow**, which can be purchased online at Juverest.com. This is a special pillow designed by a board-certified plastic surgeon from Las Vegas to prevent the formation of sleep wrinkles. Once you get over the fact that it's shaped like the thick molded Styrofoam that's used to pack electronics and computer equipment and you decide to use it anyway, it may actually work well for you. It has a special cradle for your head if you're a back sleeper and face support for side sleepers, leaving the face completely un-creased throughout the night. Now, that's real beauty sleep!

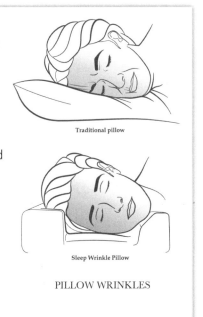

Traditional pillow

Sleep Wrinkle Pillow

PILLOW WRINKLES

Q: *If collagen is the problem, should I try collagen cream?*
Not unless you like to spend money for no good reason. Collagen creams make a lot of exciting claims that sound too good to be true, and they are. Skin is made from collagen, and that collagen degrades and breaks down over time. Imagine a sturdy little log cabin. Over the years, when subjected to the elements and the wear and tear of people living in and around it, the cabin ages. The logs become chipped, weathered, and splintered. This is what happens to your skin.

It may seem logical that if your skin is losing collagen, rubbing collagen on your face would help the problem, but unfortunately, the collagen molecule is too large to penetrate the skin. You are simply placing collagen on the surface, and this cannot change the skin's structure. The only thing collagen creams really do is moisturize your skin, which can make it look younger for a couple of hours, but you can do that for a lot less money than you will spend on a high-end collagen cream.

To fix an aging log cabin, you might have to deconstruct it and replace a few logs. Fortunately, there are also ways to get inside the skin and actually rejuvenate collagen, using procedures like laser treatments, chemical peels, and even injectable fillers. I'll talk more about these treatments later in this book.

Q. *I've heard that Preparation H will get rid of my undereye bags. Sweet! I didn't think anything would work to get rid of those!*

Don't get too excited about slathering your face with hemorrhoid ointment just yet. This is an urban legend that has been out there for a long time. "Celebrity secret to get rid of undereye bags before red carpet event!" Unfortunately, the active ingredient that supposedly worked to eliminate undereye bags was removed from the product years ago—at least in the United States. Some people believe that the Canadian-formulated version of Preparation H still contains a live yeast extract called Bio-Dyne, and that this ingredient is responsible for the undereye miracle. The ingredient in the U.S. formulation that replaced Bio-Dyne, phenylephrine, is a vasoconstrictor and may help mildly improve lower eyelid puffiness, but most people believe it doesn't work as well as Canadian Preparation H with Bio-Dyne.

However, if you want to try Preparation H (from Canada or elsewhere) under your eyes, be careful. This product is not meant to be used near the eyes, as it is intended for, shall we say, regions both lower and on the backside of the body. Don't get it in your eyes, because it could cause major irritation. In fact, if you are looking for a cream specially formulated to immediately but temporarily reduce lower eyelid puffiness, I have some great suggestions later on in the book that are very affordable and really work (see pages 125–29).

Q. *Can I change the size of my pores? They are large and I hate them.*

Pore size is determined by factors beyond your control: genetics, skin type, and age. However, you can reduce the appearance of pore size pretty easily, so you don't have to obsess about those "gaping holes" in your nose that you keep examining in the magnifying mirror. The best ways to make pores less noticeable are:

* Keep your face clean using a good cleanser. Dirty pores look bigger. Cleansers containing salicylic acid are good at cleaning out pores and preventing them from getting clogged.

* Follow cleansing with an exfoliating product a few days a week. Look for one containing alpha-hydroxy acid (AHA). I'll talk more about exfoliating later in this book.

* Periodic chemical peels can also keep pores looking smaller. I'll talk more about these later, too.

Q. *Does my car window protect me from UV radiation? Or can I get a tan in the car?*

Car windows block UVB rays, which cause the skin to tan and burn, but not UVA rays, which can cause sun damage, wrinkles, and even skin cancer.[1] If you drive a lot, check out your left hand and arm and the left side of your face. I bet you will notice more dark spots and sun damage on the left side than on the right side. This is very common. And it doesn't matter whether you drive a Lexus, a RAV4, or even an old Gremlin. Later in this book, I'll tell you exactly what to do about this problem.

Q: *What about clothing, like hats and T-shirts? Those will protect me from the sun, right?*

Hats and T-shirts seem like total protection, but it turns out that clothing isn't as effective at blocking UV rays as we once thought. T-shirts provide the protection of a sunscreen with an SPF of just 5 to 10, and this protection is decreased if the shirt is wet.[2] This is not nearly enough to protect our skin for longer than a few minutes. For this reason, you should put sunscreen on your face and body even if you are covered up. There is, however, commercially available clothing that is specially manufactured to provide sun protection. It can be a reasonable option for you if you don't want to slather sunblock over your entire body. Instead of being labeled with an SPF, its ability to block the sun's rays is measured as UPF (ultraviolet protection factor). Look for clothing that has a UPF of at least 50. Some prominent brands include **Solumbra**, **Coolibar**, and **Solartex**. Don't look for a UPF on your regular clothes, though. It's reported only for clothing that is specially designed to protect your skin from the sun.

Q: *I've read that sunlight is actually good for you because it creates vitamin D, and most people are vitamin D deficient because of sunscreen. I've also heard some of these people saying that sunlight is "natural" and humans are meant to be exposed to it. Should I be tanning to get my vitamin D level up, or should I be more "natural"?*

It's true that vitamin D is essential for the health and growth of bones and for other important processes in the body. It is also true that the skin produces vitamin D when exposed to sunlight. We all need vitamin D, and it is difficult to get enough from food. However, too much sun exposure really does damage your skin and causes premature aging, wrinkles, and skin cancer. This is an indisputable fact. The good news is that you can get your skin to produce vitamin D with very minimal sun exposure. The sunlight you get through your car window or walking around outside during the day is typically all you need, about ten to fifteen minutes each day.

If you are worried that you don't have enough vitamin D, get tested. It is easy for your doctor to do a vitamin D test at your next appointment. Just ask. If you do have low vitamin D, the best solution isn't to lie out in your bikini slathered in baby oil (it's dangerous—and *so* 1980s). Instead, take a vitamin D supplement. A good starting dose in cases of deficiency is 600–800 IU per day, but your doctor can give you more specific advice for your individual needs.

Q: *If I want the benefits of an ingredient, then I will get them as long as the ingredient is listed on my product's label. Because they can't lie to me, right?*
Actually, although a company technically cannot lie on the packaging, they can include an ingredient in such a small amount that it doesn't actually have any effect, and still advertise that the product contains that ingredient (because technically, it does). Sneaky, right? When a product contains something the FDA classifies as a drug (such as tretinoin) as opposed to a supplement (such as vitamin C) or a cosmetic (such as moisturizer), it must have a separate list called "active ingredients" for the drug ingredients. Everything else goes on a list called "inactive ingredients." However, even an item on an active ingredients list isn't necessarily present in therapeutic amounts.

Just as with food products, ingredients in skin-care and other personal-care products are listed in order of how much of that ingredient the product contains. The first ingredient is the most prevalent. The last ingredient may be there only in minuscule amounts. The product doesn't actually have to tell you how much of each ingredient it contains, although some products use this as a selling point, telling you they have X number of micrograms or whatever measure of a particular ingredient, so you know for sure it is a therapeutic dose. Or they tell you the amount but assume you probably don't know what a therapeutic dose really is. In general, if you want the benefits of a particular ingredient, make sure it is listed in the first half of the ingredients list. If it's in the second half, it is probably present in amounts too small to be effective.

Q: *Do hand sanitizers dry out and age my hands more than soap?*
Hand sanitizers usually contain alcohol, and alcohol does have a drying effect on the skin. However, alcohol is actually less drying on your skin than soap and water, which strip your hands of essential natural moisturizing oils even more than hand sanitizers do. If you have a job that requires clean hands (if you are a health-care professional, for example), it's better to use hand sanitizer when appropriate rather than constantly washing your hands with soap and water. Your skin will thank you and your hands will look better.

However, keep in mind that while hand sanitizer kills germs, it does not remove actual dirt from your hands. If you have been changing a diaper or handling food or gardening, wash your hands with soap and water afterward. Hand sanitizer is not enough. It is especially not "poop-worthy."

Q. *It seems like my leg/underarm/beard hair grows back thicker after I shave it. Is this true?*

When I was in high school, I held off shaving for as long as I could, since I heard that once you start shaving hair, it grows back even thicker than before. I spent at least two years of high school with nasty, scraggly patches of recently sprouted hair on my chin and upper lip. My friends called me "Catfish Youn." No wonder I couldn't get dates. Unfortunately, I endured this torture for nothing.

For some reason, even twenty-five years later, people continue to believe hair grows back thicker after it's shaved. But it is just not true. There is nothing about shaving a hair in the middle of its shaft that signals the body to change the quality, thickness, or anything else about the hair. Not even the length. Some people think that shaving triggers the hair to start growing again, but this isn't how hair growth works. Hair grows to a certain length, hangs out for a while, then drops off the body. If you shave the dormant hairs, eventually they will fall out. If you shave the hairs that are still growing, they will continue to grow, and then stop when they get to their designated length, after which they will go dormant and then fall out. This is the hair life cycle.

However, hair does *look* thicker when you shave, because the base of the hair shaft is thicker than the tip of the hair shaft. When you lop off the skinny part of the hair, the thicker part grows out and feels stubbly and less pliable than it did when you could feel only the soft, thin end of the natural hair. It's still the same hair of the same diameter, however, so shave away. You're not going to transform into a caveman. Or a catfish.

Q. *I have some spider veins and now even a few varicose veins. Yikes! Is this because I always cross my legs when I sit?*

Fear not. There are many causes for spider and varicose veins, but crossing your legs isn't one of them. The real causes of varicose veins are genetics, standing for long periods of time day after day (especially if you have a genetic propensity to develop them), and pregnancy. If you like how your legs look when you cross them, then knock yourself out. It's not going to make the vein situation any worse (and there are ways to fix these veins, which I'll talk about later in this book).

Q. *Should I get a "lunchtime facelift"? Isn't that a great alternative to a more drastic surgery?*

Trendy lunchtime facelifts sound appealing. Fancy commercials claim they can take ten years off your face in an hour, with no recovery time. However, I do not recommend these procedures. In fact, I suggest you run in the opposite direction. Lunchtime facelifts are basically a commoditization of plastic surgery procedures by aggressive businesspeople and profit-motivated doctors. Here is the business model:

* Hire a bunch of bargain-basement doctors to do surgery on the cheap.

* Teach them to do one or two simple cosmetic procedures as quickly as possible.

* Create infomercials and buy ads that claim these simple procedures are "revolutionary."

* Show deceptive photos. "Before" photos show patients looking miserable, with no makeup, under bad lighting. "After" photos have them holding their heads high to stretch out their necks, sporting professional makeup, and looking happy. We would all look transformed under these conditions, surgery or no surgery. (The photos could also show the results of more aggressive plastic surgery and not the lunchtime facelift procedures at all—because who is checking to be sure? Nobody.)

* Hire professional salespeople to hard-sell to patients. These salespeople are trained to convince potential clients that they need this procedure and they need it now, and if they don't do it soon, they will have to pay much more later. Pay these salespeople hefty commissions to sign up people for surgery.

* Set up bogus websites full of fake testimonials about how great the lunchtime facelift procedure is.

* Hire a team of attorneys to shut down anyone who tries to investigate the company or expose the truth about the company.

* Rake in the profits.

Be aware that any cosmetic surgery is only as good as the doctor or surgeon who performs it, and doctors who do lunchtime facelifts are not usually doctors I would want working on me, or you. There is a reason why reputable, board-certified plastic surgeons like myself do not perform lunchtime facelifts. They do not work. If it sounds too good to be true, it probably is. If you need plastic surgery, do your research and work with a reputable professional, not a company that is less interested in doing the job correctly and safely than in making a quick buck by cutting corners (on your face!).

Q: *Scars are signs of bad plastic surgery, right? If the plastic surgeon is really a good plastic surgeon, shouldn't my scars eventually disappear?*

If only we could perform magic, we would. However, there is no such thing as an invisible or completely disappearing scar. After even a short surgery that requires an incision, a scar is created. The body then begins to heal the scar, for twenty-four hours a day, seven days a week, four weeks a month, for six or even up to twelve months. At that time, the scar will be mature and you will know how it's going to look pretty much for the rest of your life. The plastic surgeon has very little control over this process. Scars are permanent, and the way they heal has a lot to do with aftercare and your individual body and skin. Will the scar get infected? Are you picking at it? Does your skin heal quickly or slowly? These and many other considerations affect wound healing. You can try to alter your body's healing response by using a good silicone-based scar cream or undergoing laser treatments or steroid injections to minimize scarring, but even if you do all of these things, your body might still create a thicker, more unsightly scar than someone else's body. It might also create a scar that becomes barely noticeable over time.

What your surgeon should be able to tell you is whether the scar will have suture tracks (the tiny dot-like scars on both sides of a scar that can result if sutures are left in too long), whether the scar will look jagged, and whether it will look bunched up. But that's about all we can tell. However, good surgeons do have a few tricks up their sleeves, like the best places to put incisions so scars are less noticeable. Beyond that, a scar is a scar and a necessary part of any plastic surgery that requires an incision.

One last thing: I've noticed over the last fifteen years that older people (typically older than sixty) tend to scar much better than younger people. Their scars are thinner and lighter and have a much lower tendency to thicken and look unsightly. This may be due to the collagen in their skin being thinner and less likely to overgrow and bunch up in the healing process. I find the people who scar the worst are in their twenties to their forties. This is one good thing about getting older!

Q: *I've heard that liposuctioned fat comes back in a different place, and/or in a weird, lumpy shape. Is this true?*

This is controversial, but personally, I think it sounds silly. I (and many of my plastic surgeon colleagues) have always believed and informed our patients that liposuctioned fat will not return to another area. If I suck fat out of your thighs, it's not going to reappear on your upper arms.

However, in 2011, a study was performed at the University of Colorado that suggested this could actually happen.[3] The study was performed on thirty-two volunteers, and it found that after liposuction of the thighs, strange excess pockets of fat appeared on the trunk and even the arms, as if the liposuctioned fat had somehow returned to a different location. I call it the "Popeye Effect." However, another, larger study on 301 patients a year later refuted the findings, suggesting that perhaps there was a problem with the original, much smaller study.[4]

So what is the truth? Does liposuctioned fat come back? Does it trigger some kind of reaction in the body that causes the remaining existing fat to expand in size? All I can tell you is that over the past ten years, I've performed liposuction on at least two hundred people per year, totaling about two thousand patients. I've honestly had only one patient tell me the fat I removed came back. However, she admitted that this happened after she gained a lot of weight gorging on food over the holidays. As a doctor, I have to say that clearly, the old fat hadn't come back. Her lapse into bad lifestyle habits had caused her remaining fat to expand. I have never had a patient tell me that the fat removed from one area came back in a different area. Never.

Q: *I heard that if I get breast implants my breasts won't droop as I get older. Is this true?*

No! It's completely false. Breast implants act as weights in your breasts. Gravity pulls on them, day in and day out. The bigger they are, the heavier they are and the more quickly they will sag. It's simple physics. The only exception to this is Pamela Anderson. Her breasts are massive, and it's even been rumored that her breast implants are stacked, meaning there is more than one implant in each breast. Still, even over fifteen years after she left *Baywatch*, her breasts look as perky as ever. They seem to defy gravity. Putting Pam and her amazing hovering breasts aside, there are some actions you can take (and your surgeon can take) if you have breast implants to prevent them from sagging as quickly as they might otherwise. Wear a supportive bra with underwire during the day. Wear a sports bra when you work out. And probably most important of all: If you do decide that you have to have breast implants, don't go any larger than necessary to make you feel balanced.

These are the myths and truths I encounter day after day in my practice. Now that we've set the record straight, I bet you want to get right down to business. In the next section, we'll talk about aging, what it does to your skin, and the easy routines and lifestyle changes you can make to get the most out of your natural beauty and youthful internal processes. Are you ready to start looking better today? Read on.

3 | YOUR SKIN, YOUR AGE, YOUR BEAUTY

In some ways, beauty really is skin-deep, and no part of your body shows aging quite as obviously and dramatically as your skin. Skin issues of all kinds plague many of my patients, especially issues that cause people to look older. It's usually the first thing people ask me about, and yet I find that most people don't understand how skin is constructed, how it ages, why it ages, and what they can do about it.

Maybe you are desperate to look younger and you will try just about anything, or maybe you don't like your wrinkles and you'd rather not get any more of them, but you don't think there's much you can do if you don't want plastic surgery. Fortunately, you are wrong. You do not have to be at the mercy of your skin. There are many tricks, techniques, products, and procedures that target everything from wrinkles to age spots to sagging jowls and nasolabial folds, and you won't have to go under the knife to try them. I've seen noticeable, often dramatic differences in the skin quality and appearance of my patients. I've seen them appear to grow younger before my eyes. This can be you. Are you ready to look younger than you do right now?

SKIN BASICS

You've got about twenty square feet of skin on your body, and it has a big job to do. It keeps dirt and pathogens out of your insides, and it excretes oil through tiny holes called pores to keep your skin protected and moisturized. Your skin can even soak up medicine and other substances, like the hormones in a birth control patch or the nicotine in a nicotine patch. The skin is technically your largest organ, even though it doesn't look like an organ. It's also more complex than it appears.

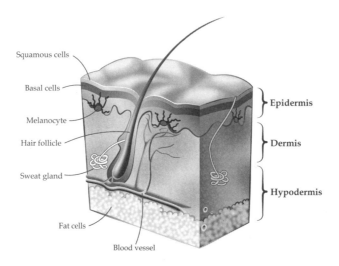

Squamous cells
Basal cells
Melanocyte
Hair follicle
Sweat gland
Fat cells
Blood vessel
Epidermis
Dermis
Hypodermis

UNDERSTANDING SKIN ANATOMY

Skin contains three layers:

The Epidermis

Your epidermis is showing! This is the fancy name for your skin, specifically the outer layer of skin that you see. Because it is the layer visible to the world (and in the mirror), this is where your efforts at skin care will show up most dramatically.

Depending on what's going on with your epidermis, your skin can look plump, moist, and youthful or thin, dry, and wrinkled. The very top layer of the epidermis is mostly dead skin cells, and the bottom layer is the basal cells, which divide. As the new basal cells divide, they move up toward the surface, and eventually die and slough off. All day we are sloughing dead skin cells, leaving them in our mattresses, on our clothing, and even, if you haven't bathed in a few days, as a ring around the tub! This constant turnover slows down as you get older, and also with exposure to sun and environmental toxins. This causes the layer of older dead cells to clump and build up, causing you to look flaky, dull, rough, and, frankly, older. This is why exfoliating treatments make you look younger—they get rid of the top layer of the oldest dead skin cells and expose the younger, newer cells.

The other thing the epidermis contains is melanocytes. These are the cells that create melanin, which is the pigment that gives your skin its unique color. Melanin protects you from sun damage, darkening to be more protective when you are exposed to the sun. Yes, a suntan is really your body's reaction to shield you from the damaging rays. As you age, the melanocytes can become more irregular in their production of pigment, which causes age spots and melasma (a condition in which sun exposure or hormone changes cause dark patches of skin on the face). Even though the epidermis turns all its skin cells over every six to eight weeks, you don't get a newborn-baby face every two months, unfortunately. The mechanisms that create the new cells age and get damaged, and the age spots and flaky patches you have can remain or keep coming back. However, don't be discouraged. The lifestyle measures and treatment that I'll soon introduce to you can drastically improve your skin's look, color, plumpness, and even tone.

The Dermis

The dermis is a thicker layer beneath the epidermis. You don't see this layer, but it's pretty busy under there. The dermis contains strong connective tissue to give the thinner epidermis support. It's mostly made out of collagen, elastin, and hyaluronic acid.

Collagen is what most of the skin is made out of, which is why you see all those skin-care products that contain collagen. Collagen fibers are strong protein fibers that are organized in parallel bands. They are like the bricks of your skin that are held together by elastin, which is like the mortar. We have the most collagen when we are children. Collagen production slows down in the teen years, holds constant through our twenties and thirties, and then starts to decline, which is one major reason why you will start to notice signs of aging in your thirties. The quality of your collagen determines how tight your skin looks and feels. When it becomes weakened, or those parallel bands of collagen become frayed and damaged by aging, sun exposure, and other trauma, your skin will begin to look more wrinkled, saggy, and old.

Elastin is what gives skin its elastic nature. When you pull on your skin, it bounces back to its original position. Hyaluronic acid is a sugar that binds water and attracts moisture. This is what makes your skin look moist and plump. The main reason young skin looks so young is because it's plumped up with lots of collagen, elastin, and hyaluronic acid, and the reason faces look older as they age is because all of these components decrease with age. Skin gets less plump and juicy, and so it looks thinner, drier, saggier, and more wrinkled. This is why many skin-care products also contain elastin and hyaluronic acid. So, do skin-care products containing the three main elements of skin—collagen, elastin, and hyaluronic acid—actually restore these to your skin? That depends on the delivery system. I'll talk more about this later in this chapter and in the next chapter.

The dermis also contains a few other things: fibroblasts that produce collagen and elastin, hair follicles, sweat glands, and sebaceous glands, which produce an oily-ish, waxy substance called sebum for skin lubrication. Overactive sebaceous glands can cause acne, because they are producing too much sebum, which bacteria can feed on, causing pimples.

The Hypodermis

This is the deepest layer of skin, and the fattest layer. In fact, it contains fat and connective tissue, and it overlays your muscle and bone. It also contains fibroblasts and macrophages, but its primary purpose is for fat storage. This is where our dreaded cellulite lives. We'll talk more about cellulite and what you can do about it in chapter 8.

AGING AND YOUR SKIN

Why does aging change your skin, and why oh why can't it just stay the same as it was when you were young, before you ever had a pimple, before you were exposed to pollution or thought tanning was a great idea? The reason is that life quite literally happens to you, and your skin is the primary barrier between you and the world. It is your shield, and it gets battered by time and life experience. Women typically begin to show the first signs of aging in their mid-twenties, while men begin to show the first signs about five years later, only because they have thicker skin. Their shields are a bit thicker, but aging happens to us all eventually.

Aging happens due to two different kinds of influences: intrinsic and extrinsic. You can't do much about intrinsic aging. It is caused by your genetics, such as a propensity to stay looking younger longer or to get wrinkles at a younger age. One celebrity who appears to have inherited a slow intrinsic aging process is Kate Hudson. Her mom, Goldie Hawn, didn't seem to age for decades, and now Kate looks as if she's following in her footsteps. Intrinsic aging is also caused by your ethnicity. Different ethnic skin types withstand aging better or worse than others. Dr. Travis Stork, host of the syndicated show *The Doctors,* once asked me how my skin was so smooth and wrinkle free. I answered him honestly that it was a combination of TV makeup and my ethnicity!

Intrinsic aging can also be caused by certain disease conditions, which can prematurely age your skin. An extreme example of this is the genetic disorder progeria, or the anti–Benjamin Button syndrome, where the affected person's body ages incredibly quickly. You can't change your genetics, your ethnicity, or arguably your disease state. However, you can definitely do something about extrinsic aging.

Extrinsic aging is caused by factors that you can control, and it is the main focus of this book. Fortunately, extrinsic aging is a major part of aging, so while you can't turn the clock back forever, you can definitely slow it down pretty significantly. There are four major factors that cause extrinsic aging:

1. **Sun damage.** Excess ultraviolet radiation is the absolute worst thing you can expose your skin to if you want to keep it looking young. You probably already know that ultraviolet radiation increases your risk of skin cancer. However, it also has a striking effect on aging. All you have to do to determine whether ultraviolet light has already aged you beyond how you would age without exposure is to compare the skin on a part of your body that gets a lot of sun, like your face or your arms, with parts of your body that get almost no sun, like your butt cheeks. Check out your butt cheeks. (I won't look.) Notice how nice and smooth they are? They don't have age spots or wrinkles, and while they might have a few cellulite dimples or not be the exact size or shape you would prefer, the skin itself is looking pretty good, wouldn't you say? Imagine how young you would look if your facial skin and the skin on your hands and forearms looked like the skin on your butt. Clearly, being called a butt-face is really a compliment!

2. **Smoking.** Smoking is second only to UV radiation in its aging effects on the skin. Smoking constricts the blood vessels, which decreases blood supply to your skin. It also dehydrates your skin, increases free-radical damage, and has been linked to an increased risk of skin cancer.[5] One study showed that the risk of developing severe wrinkles was three times higher in smokers than in nonsmokers.[6] Another demonstrated that heavy smokers were 4.7 times more likely to be wrinkled than nonsmokers.[7] That's reason enough to throw that pack of cigarettes in the trash!

3. **Eating poorly.** You know it's not healthy for your insides, but did you know that poor dietary choices can make visible differences in your skin? Sugar in particular is a skin wrecker, as it causes aging by increasing inflammation and glycation. Eating the right kinds of fats can actually help you look younger, however. I'll talk much more about eating for younger skin in chapter 5.

4. **Drinking too much alcohol.** Excessive alcohol consumption is bad for you in all kinds of ways, and one of those ways is by aging your skin prematurely. Alcohol dehydrates your skin and causes some people to have a flushing reaction. Repeated flushing can result in a ruddy complexion, and I don't mean that healthy glow you get when you've been on a hike. I mean the kind caused by tiny broken blood vessels that show up as splotchy red patches all over your face. It's not pretty. Too much alcohol can also keep you from other healthy habits, like eating well, and can encourage other unhealthy

habits, like smoking. Sit out on the beach in the sun with a cigarette and a cocktail, and you've got a recipe for overnight aging.

The effects that these four factors have on skin aren't just about dehydration and blood vessel constriction or swelling. They're also about free radicals. In fact, a significant amount of aging in the body is caused by free radicals, and you have the power to greatly minimize these effects.

Free radicals are damaged oxygen molecules that are missing at least one electron. To remedy the problem, they attach to healthy cells and steal their electrons, damaging the cells or causing them to malfunction. This can cause all sorts of problems, from cell structure damage to DNA damage. Free radicals are by-products of the body's various processes, like digestion, and they should be present in amounts the body can easily handle. However, when you add in extrinsic factors like UV exposure, smoking, a poor diet, alcohol, and the effects of toxins like pollution, pesticides, automobile exhaust, and environmental chemicals, and especially when you have more than one of these operating on the body at one time, free radicals can become too numerous.

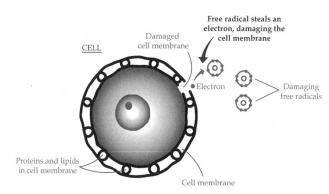

FREE RADICALS

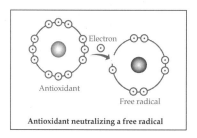

NEUTRALIZING FREE RADICALS

When this happens, the body enters a state of oxidative stress, where it cannot fend off all the free-radical damage on its own. Free radicals then begin to cause visible damage. One type is a breakdown in collagen and elastin, making the skin looser, more wrinkled, and thinner. As we age, collagen production slows down, so we don't replace the collagen that gets broken down as quickly. Eventually, we hardly replace it at all.

This is why the best antiaging treatments address free radicals in their formulations. First on the list: antioxidants. Antioxidants fight free radicals by neutralizing them. They donate an extra electron to the free radical, essentially stopping it from scavenging electrons from other cells. Your body naturally produces antioxidants, but if you add more through diet (see chapter 5) and the right skin-care products, you can help your body immensely. Antioxidants are like the cavalry sweeping in to fight off the free-radical onslaught. See the next chapter for more specific information about antioxidant products.

Fountain of Youth

If you are a person with darker skin, you have an aging advantage. Darker skin tends to be thicker and produce more oil than lighter skin. That means there is more collagen, and the skin is more resistant to aging and wrinkling. More oil means more natural moisture, so the skin doesn't look as dry and dull as lighter skin can. You can see it for yourself if you compare celebrities of similar ages over thirty who have light versus dark skin. Those with dark skin almost always look younger, and the difference is more pronounced with increasing age. Check out Oprah Winfrey and her buddy Gayle King. Both are in their sixties, have had no obvious plastic surgeries, and look like they're in their forties!

ANTIAGING ATTACK

Now that you know what's happening to age your skin, let's get down to business and attack aging where it starts: on your face, in the form of wrinkles, fine lines, and age spots. In the next chapter, we'll talk more about lifestyle issues, specifically diet, but first I want to focus on the products, procedures, and even natural therapies that I have seen make a real difference in the appearance of my patients' skin. I'll also clue you in to which products, techniques, and procedures probably won't do what they claim, so you can save your time and money for the strategies that really work.

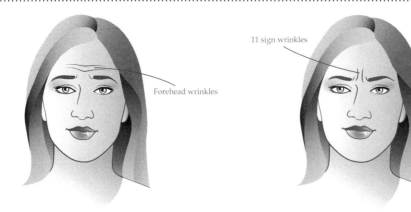

Forehead wrinkles

11 sign wrinkles

Forehead Wrinkles

Little kids have smooth foreheads because they haven't spent years raising their eyebrows and scrunching up their foreheads. Forehead wrinkles primarily consist of two types: the horizontal lines across the forehead that you get when you raise your eyebrows, which are caused by the contraction of the frontalis muscles; and the little vertical lines between your eyebrows, called the 11 sign, which are caused when you furrow your brows to make that stern expression while scolding your kids or the dog. The 11 sign is, hands down, the most common cosmetic complaint I see in my office. Of all the patients who come in to look younger, at least 60 percent of them complain about their 11 signs. As far as aging, it's endemic! If you are one of the few (very few!) who are over forty and don't have an 11 sign, be very thankful. For the rest: After years of creasing your forehead horizontally and vertically, those creases are going to stick.

These are also called dynamic lines, because they are caused by muscle movement. The best way to treat dynamic lines like forehead wrinkles and the 11 sign is to stop the muscles from contracting and making these wrinkles. Here are my recommendations:

Botox: There is no question that Botox is the most effective way to reduce wrinkles in the forehead and between the eyebrows. In fact, it's FDA-approved for treatment of lines between the eyebrows. However, people worry about Botox. They connect it with a lot of scary things: frozen foreheads, drooping mouths, perma-smiles, and even death from black-market Botox. I hate to say it, but many of these problems have occurred. Those fears have a basis, but they needn't be a problem for you if you choose the right doctor.

I admit Botox sounds scary when you know what it really is. Botox is the trade name for botulinum toxin, a neurotoxin created by the bacterium *Clostridium botulinum.*

Botulinum toxin is one of the most dangerous poisons in the world, and small to moderate amounts that are injected or inhaled can kill a person. So how is it that Botox is now the number one cosmetic treatment in the world, with nearly 4 million Americans undergoing Botox injections in 2014, according to the American Society for Aesthetic Plastic Surgery? The difference is in dosage. While a small amount of botulinum toxin can kill you, the minuscule amounts used in Botox injections will not harm you at all. They will paralyze only the immediate area where the toxin is injected, and that's good news for you (and bad news for your wrinkles). Botulinum toxin was first used to effectively treat spastic muscle disorders of the eyes and eyelids, otherwise known as strabismus and blepharospasm. Botulinum toxin, when used in minute amounts, was found to be very effective at relaxing these spastic muscles, thereby improving the disorders. This led two enterprising dermatologists from Canada, Drs. J. A. and J. D. Carruthers (a married couple), to wonder: If it's good enough to weaken muscles in the eyes and eyelids, why can't it be good enough to weaken the muscles of the face that cause wrinkles?

They decided to test the botulinum toxin's effects on the wrinkle-causing muscles in the face, and they discovered that when the tiniest quantities of botulinum toxin were injected into the muscles that caused wrinkles in the glabella (that is, the vertical frown lines between the eyebrows and above the nose, otherwise known as the "11 sign"), they caused the muscles to weaken, resulting in a temporary smoothing of wrinkles. And voila! Botox was born.

Now Botox is one of the favorite and most effective antiaging treatments available. It is used in minute quantities and is injected into the muscles that create these wrinkles. Within a week or two, these muscles weaken and even become temporarily paralyzed. This causes the muscles and the wrinkles to relax and look smoother. Botox typically wears off within three to four months, after which time it needs to be repeated. Otherwise, the wrinkles return like they were before. You can also try one of Botox's competitors, such as **Dysport**. Results with Dysport are very similar to results with Botox.

People worry about Botox because they know it is a toxin. It even sounds a little scary to those who aren't familiar with it. However, Botox is extremely safe, and in the hands of a board-certified plastic surgeon or dermatologist, you are extremely likely to have excellent results. Prior to Botox, plastic surgeons and dermatologists used lasers and chemical peels to improve forehead wrinkles. The results were minimal at best, since the wrinkles are caused by muscles, and these treatments affect only the skin on top of the muscles.

If you're considering Botox but are nervous that the treatment might make you look like a mannequin, a Disney cartoon, or even worse, a Real Housewife of Beverly Hills, then start small. Try treating either your crow's-feet or the 11 sign. If your doctor treats one of these areas conservatively, it's very unlikely you will look strange or "done." Give yourself a couple of weeks after the treatment to get used to the results. If you're happy with them (which almost everyone is), then return to treat another area (or two). Just be careful when getting your forehead Botoxed. When Botox is improperly injected into the forehead, it can cause the dreaded "frozen forehead" appearance where your eyebrows don't move. Or, even worse, you can get Frozen Forehead's horrible cousin, Evil Eyebrow. This is when your brows become overly arched, making you look like the cartoon version of *Sleeping Beauty*'s wicked Maleficent.

Before we finish covering Botox, here is a question: What do Botox treatments have in common with smoking cigarettes and drinking booze?

They're addictive.

No, not in the unhealthy way that the body becomes chemically addicted to the toxins nicotine and alcohol. Millions of people are "addicted" to the way Botox smooths their lines, reduces their wrinkles, and relaxes their stern expressions. Once you see how a conservative amount of Botox can make you look, you may become addicted, too. We have many return clients.

No-Scrunch Zone: If Botox just isn't for you, there is another way. It takes a little more effort, but it can make a difference. It is possible to train your muscles to stop contracting so much, thereby smoothing the wrinkles of your forehead naturally. I work on this myself—unless I'm modeling these wrinkles for my patients, I try not to scrunch my forehead or between my eyebrows as much as possible.

It can be tricky to isolate small muscles in the face or elsewhere, but with a little concentration and practice, you can learn to do it. Remember when you first learned to raise your eyebrows, flare your nostrils, or wiggle your ears? That's facial muscle control. In acting classes, they teach the minute control of facial muscles to help actors master various expressions. If they can do it, so can you. However, it's not easy, so here are some tricks that can help you with your facial muscle training:

* Put tape over your forehead during the evening and while you sleep. This essentially keeps the skin smooth, and if you try to scrunch your face, you will feel the tape and be reminded not to do it. Some people even scrunch their foreheads while they sleep, so putting tape on your forehead while you sleep can help prevent this from happening.

* There is a commercially available product that works in a way similar to the tape. **Frownies** are patches you wear over your wrinkles that actually splint the wrinkle and

prevent your skin from contracting and creasing, or at least call your attention to it so it feels uncomfortable when you do it. The makers claim that Frownies will train your muscles at night to prevent them from contracting during the day. It makes sense in theory and would probably be helpful for those willing to put in the effort to also be more aware of their facial wrinkling habits.

I wish I could tell you that there was a magic cream that would eliminate forehead creases without any other effort, but like the lasers and chemical peels doctors used to try, creams really affect only the skin and do not impact the muscle underneath. Because the muscle is the issue with this particular type of wrinkling, the muscle has to be the point of treatment.

Insider Tip

Professional makeup artists and aestheticians have secrets, and knowing their philosophy can help you apply your own makeup more effectively so you look better and younger. One of the most important things I've learned from these professionals is that most cosmetic effort should go into enhancing your assets rather than trying to cover up or camouflage your perceived flaws. If you aren't sure how to do this, I definitely recommend getting a professional consultation.

Even if you think you know best how to do your own makeup, open your mind to updated advice. You don't have to go to a fancy makeup boutique where you know you will be pressured to spend hundreds of dollars. Instead, go to your local department store's makeup counter. Analyze the makeup artist salespeople from afar. When you find one whose makeup you like, approach her. Let her know you are interested in some ideas about how to do your makeup differently and ask her if she could show you how she does hers. Then you can either buy the makeup she recommends or, if you are strapped for cash, get a $10 lipstick and then head to the drugstore to get similar products at a lower price.

Fine Lines

If you've had a thirtieth birthday, you've probably had this experience: You wake up, you look in the mirror, and there they are. You hadn't really noticed them before, because you were in your twenties. Now that you are thirty, you see them, and they are only going to get worse: those fine lines forming on your face. Fine lines add a subtle age to your face, even if they are not obvious creases. The difference between a young face and a middle-aged face is largely about fine lines. Fine lines are caused by a combination of factors, including sun damage, environmental toxins, dry skin, loss of collagen and elastin, and skin-muscle interactions. They are the inevitable result of aging and life in the world, and there are no surgical treatments that will erase them. However, there are some nonsurgical treatments that can make them look much less noticeable, and even eliminate some or most of them, depending on how many you have.

I once had a patient drive five hours to see me for a consultation on a facelift. Immediately upon my entrance into the exam room, she pulled out a large wad of bills and said, "I've been saving for years for my facelift. Just tell me where and when you can do it." I asked her what was bothering her about her face and what specifically she wanted to improve. She pointed to fine lines under her eyes, around her mouth, and on the sides of her face. I informed her that no facelift, no actual surgery, can remove fine lines. There is nothing I can do with a scalpel to get rid of them! We started her on the right skin-care products and signed her up for a series of chemical peels. Then I instructed her to use the rest of the money she'd saved (several thousand dollars) on a dream vacation instead. A week of pure relaxation is another excellent way to make your face look younger, because it melts away stress, which makes you crease your face into wrinkles. This is hard to do while lying on a beach under an umbrella with a fruity drink!

But back to those fine lines. Remember the structure of the skin: The epidermis is the top layer that generates skin cells. They move up toward the surface, die, and eventually fall off. As these cells build up, fine lines can become more noticeable, because dry, flaky skin shows off fine lines. This is why one of the best treatments for fine lines is exfoliation, or removal of the upper layers of the skin. This can cause the skin to look smoother and reduce the appearance of fine lines, because you will be sloughing off the dry dead cells and revealing the younger cells beneath. You can do this at home, but there are more aggressive ways of exfoliating in a medical setting.

CO_2 Lasers: The most aggressive way of doing this is with the old-fashioned CO_2 laser. The problem with this laser is that it is ablative, meaning it literally burns off the entire upper layer of skin. This leaves people not only feeling like burn patients but sporting redness and even oozing. The procedure is painful and the recovery time is significant.

The newer CO_2 treatments are fractional, meaning instead of burning all the skin, they burn only a fraction of the skin. That may still sound harsh, but the fractional lasers are now the standard of care for aggressive treatment of fine lines and wrinkles. These lasers come in many different brands and names, such as **Fraxel**, **Active FX**, and **Deep FX**, to name a few. The downtime also varies, with some aggressive treatments necessitating a week or more to recover from them.

Sometimes, depending on how aggressive the laser is, you may need a sedative or light anesthetic to be able to tolerate the actual treatment. These laser treatments can be quite costly (in the thousands of dollars), as you are typically paying for the doctor's time in addition to the cost of leasing the laser. Fractional lasers typically cost a plastic surgeon upward of $100,000 to purchase, and the cost is therefore passed on to the patient (you).

Chemical Peels: Chemical peels are another procedure you've probably heard about. They are another way to effectively exfoliate the skin. Chemical peels come in many different types and strengths. In general, however, the more aggressive the peel, the better the results, but the longer the recovery time.

Chemical peels are typically more affordable than laser treatments because the cost of the supplies needed to perform a chemical peel can be as low as $10. Compared to the cost of purchasing and operating a laser, this is a significant difference that should be passed on to you. For that reason alone, chemical peels can be considered a cost-effective alternative to fractional laser treatments. Still, aggressive chemical peels can easily cost in the upper hundreds of dollars.

The most aggressive and effective chemical peel, the **phenol peel**, must be done under the care of a vigilant plastic surgeon or dermatologist, because the acid can create cardiac arrhythmias if overapplied. Call me a scaredy-cat, but because of the potential heart issues, I'm afraid to perform these. Not surprisingly, like the old ablative CO_2 lasers, the phenol peel is gradually going out of favor, as doctors and patients are opting for less aggressive treatments to exfoliate the skin.

In my office, I perform quite a few moderate-depth chemical peels. Although not as strong or as effective as the deeper phenol peel, these are more easily tolerated, are safer, and can get nice results, especially if repeated. My current favorite is the **ZO Controlled Depth Peel**, which uses a blue dye to create a more even, effective peel. Patients peel for a week afterward, but the recovery is completely painless. The only downside to the ZO Controlled Depth Peel is that you leave the office looking like a Smurf.

Many people undergo so-called lunchtime peels, which can have absolutely no downtime or pain. These are weaker versions of standard chemical peels, and they are great for smoothing the skin and creating some mild tightening. The results are temporary, and the peels should be repeated approximately every month to maintain their results. The lunchtime peels rarely cost more than $200, depending on the location. If these are available to you, they are a good maintenance option.

At-Home Laser Treatment: If you're more of the DIY ilk and you want to do your beauty treatments at home, there are some good options. I like a product called **Silk'n FaceFX**. This is an at-home, do-it-yourself laser that improves the look of fine lines, skin texture, and wrinkles. It takes about fifteen to twenty minutes, and you use it three times per week. The results are proven. A study showed that after eight weeks of treatment, 91 percent of users had an improvement in skin texture, and 69 percent had a reduction in fine lines and wrinkles. This is a good option for a budget-conscious person or someone who doesn't live within driving distance of a dermatologist, plastic surgeon, or med spa that provides chemical peel or laser services. It costs about $299, but I've seen advertised specials online for less, so keep an eye out.

Tretinoin (Retin-A): For a real long-term difference in fine lines, there is no better treatment than prescription-strength tretinoin, otherwise known as Retin-A. Tretinoin is scientifically proven to reduce fine lines via exfoliation and also a thickening of the dermal and epidermal layers. Results aren't immediate, however. You may see some results within two weeks, but it usually takes six to eight weeks to see any real change in fine lines. You will see a difference eventually, however, and a tube of tretinoin costs $40 to $50 with discount coupons you can find online, so it's an inexpensive option. Tretinoin is actually used as a precursor to chemical peels to prepare the skin for the peel. I tell patients that if they like what the tretinoin does for their skin, the peel will take that to the next level. Tretinoin is also an excellent remedy for acne. (See the next chapter for more information about tretinoin.) Some people are sensitive to tretinoin, but others tolerate it quite well.

Alpha-Hydroxy Acid (AHA): This product can also help with fine lines, especially when combined with tretinoin. These are fruit acids, glycolic acids, and lactic acids that exfoliate the skin, removing the upper layer of dead skin cells and indirectly stimulating new cell growth. AHAs are derived from natural sources, but be careful when combining these two exfoliating treatments, as they can be very powerful. AHAs are another good treatment for acne. See the next chapter for more detailed information about AHAs. As with Retin-A, some people are sensitive to AHAs to varying degrees, but some have great results and very little if any irritation.

Peter Thomas Roth's Un-Wrinkle Peel Pads: You can do a mild chemical peel at home. These handy pads contain a potent combination of alpha-, beta-, and even gamma-hydroxy acids to exfoliate and tighten the skin. But that's not it! This product also contains antiaging amino acids. Apply these pads once a day for great results within just a few treatments. You can purchase these online or at Sephora stores.

Dimethicone: If you're looking for an immediate change, then a powerful moisturizer can be very effective to fill in fine lines and smooth your skin. As we age, our skin dehydrates more easily, resulting in dry, wrinkled skin. Moisturizers can reverse this phenomenon and create an immediate change. Look for a moisturizer that contains hyaluronic acid, glycerin, and/or dimethicone. Dimethicone is a type of topical silicone that can immediately plump out fine lines. Dimethicone is one of the main ingredients in L'Oréal's **RevitaLift**, which is an inexpensive, easy-to-find, and effective temporary skin smoother.

Beauty Secret

Currently my favorite moisturizing skin-care line is from **Teoxane Cosmeceuticals**. Their Swiss-made serums and creams list Resilient Hyaluronic Acid as a prime ingredient. Hyaluronic acid, you may remember, is a naturally occurring moisturizer of our skin. It's also the prime ingredient in injectable wrinkle fillers like Juvederm, Restylane, and Voluma. Teoxane products are the closest thing we have to skin fillers in a tube. The products rehydrate the skin so well that it looks as if your wrinkles are literally filled in. I recently started my mom on these products (they've only recently become available in the United States), and she loves them. Teoxane is especially good for women whose skin is dry due to menopause and/or living in drier climates. I consider Teoxane products an ✱ **AGE FIX FAVORITE**.

Fruit Acids from Your Own Kitchen: If you like your beauty natural style, there are some interesting treatments you can whip up in your own kitchen that use vitamins, alpha-hydroxy acids, and other skin-boosting, beauty-enhancing ingredients:

* **Bananas** are full of vitamins A, B, and E. Mash up half a ripe banana, then apply the mash to your face. Leave it on for thirty minutes, then wash it off with warm water. Your face will feel cleaner and tighter.

* For the ultimate natural **DIY chemical peel**, combine 3 tablespoons **apple juice**, 2 tablespoons **milk**, and 1 **egg white**. Mix everything together and apply to your face.

Let it sit for fifteen minutes, then wash off with warm water. The malic acid in the apple juice and the lactic acid in the milk act as gentle exfoliants, while the albumin in the egg white has a shrink-wrap effect on the face: tightening the skin, shrinking pores, and making your face look firmer and smoother. Who knew you could get a chemical peel from apple juice?

Insider Tip

One way to disguise fine lines is through the skilled application of primer, foundation, powder, highlighter, and bronzer. You may need only one or a few of these products, or maybe you will choose to use them all, but how you put them on can make the difference between hiding fine lines and accentuating them. Here are some tips:

* Try using primer before applying makeup. This can cover blemishes and fill in fine lines before you've even applied your makeup. You can also try applying primer to your neck and chest. It can reduce the appearance of aging by covering up wrinkles and sun spots without a heavily made-up look.

* Go light and sheer with your foundation, especially as you age. Thick, heavy foundation accentuates wrinkles and creases rather than hiding them.

* Pay attention to detail. Meticulously blend so you don't have makeup lines along your jaw or covering blemishes. Foundation and concealer brushes are great tools for creating a flawless look.

* Mineral foundation that comes in a powder goes on like a liquid and can actually protect your skin, because the titanium dioxide or zinc oxide minerals shield you from sun damage. They are also less likely to cause acne. If you find that the powder looks dry on your skin, try "setting" the makeup with a spray of **Thermal Spring Water** by La Roche-Posay. This can give it a less powdery look. If this doesn't work, then it might be best to switch back to a creamy foundation.

* Match your foundation color to the color of your skin at your jawline.

* Update your powder if you haven't done so in a while. The newer powders are reflective and brightening rather than drying and cakey.

The strategic use of a highlighter can give a lifting effect to the face. Apply highlighter to areas you want to accentuate, like cheekbones, the bridge of your nose, and just under your eyebrows, to give the impression of a brow lift. Fill in the parts you want to recede with bronzer, just slightly darker than your natural skin color. Blend it all really well so there are no separation lines.

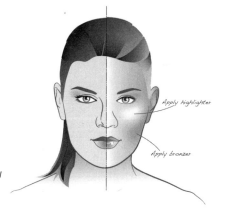

Apply highlighter

Apply bronzer

Use highlighter and bronzer to provide a lift to the cheeks.

ACNE

It's so unfair. You're dealing with fine lines at the same time you're dealing with acne! It's true—over 25 percent of women in their forties and 15 percent of women older than fifty battle adult acne, and this is the kind of acne that *doesn't* make you look like a teenager. Nope, this kind of acne tends to be cystic. Instead of that frecklelike spread of teenage redness, you get those big, pus-filled suckers in the least attractive places—smack in the middle of your chin or forehead, or around your mouth, or around the sides of your nose. You also might get blackheads—those ugly black dots caused by your pores getting clogged with oxidized (darkened) sebum. Blackheads don't get red and puffy like pimples do, but they aren't pretty, either.

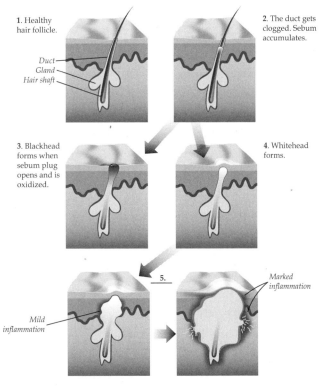

1. Healthy hair follicle.

Duct
Gland
Hair shaft

2. The duct gets clogged. Sebum accumulates.

3. Blackhead forms when sebum plug opens and is oxidized.

4. Whitehead forms.

5.

Marked inflammation

Mild inflammation

FORMATION OF ACNE

Adult acne can be caused by stress, heredity, hormone fluctuations, and even some medications, but the best treatments are, fortunately, those you can do at home. For the most effective acne eradication, try this four-step process:

1. Unclog your pores to prevent pimples and clear out blackheads.

2. Kill bacteria causing these skin infections and reduce excess oil.

3. Increase cell turnover to get younger, fresher skin faster.

4. Know how to manhandle pimples.

Here's what I recommend:

Step One: Unclog Pores

Salicylic acid is the key to unclogging pores. Use a salicylic acid–based cleanser with a strength of 1 to 2% twice a day, morning and evening. This will help scour your pores, reduce blackhead formation, and help prevent pimples from forming. Salicylic acid is a beta-hydroxy acid that comes from trees, and it is lipid soluble, so it penetrates the oily sebum plugging your pores. If you want to get serious and intimidate your acne into total submission, you can even get a salicylic acid peel in a plastic surgeon's or dermatologist's office every few weeks. This can make a big difference in keeping both blackheads and pimples at bay.

Caution!

Do not use any product containing salicylic acid if you are pregnant. Although the only proven dangers are through the oral administration of salicylic acid, most doctors recommend avoiding the topical form, too, just in case. Avoid all products containing any of the following:

* *Salicylic acid*

* *Beta-hydroxy acid* (BHA)

Another neat trick for blackheads is pore strips, like **Bioré Deep Cleansing Pore Strips**, which work to remove the sebum from pores. Pull these strips off your nose and witness hundreds of tiny piles of sebum that have been pulled right out. No more blackheads! Be very careful to pull the strips off gently if you are taking tretinoin, however. This makes your skin more delicate, and pulling the strips off roughly could inflame or even injure your skin.

Bioré strips too pricey for you? Here's a DIY trick: Apply a thin layer of **Elmer's Glue** to the skin affected by blackheads. Let it dry, then gently peel it off. The blackheads come right along with it! If that's too weird for you, you could also mix 2 teaspoons of unflavored gelatin with 2 teaspoons of milk. Warm it in the microwave for ten seconds, allow it to cool slightly, then apply it to your nose while still warm and sticky. Once it firms up, pull it off, along with the blackheads. You can do this once a week for best results. (Although these DIY treatments work, you may find the Bioré strips work better.)

Step Two: Kill Bacteria and Reduce Excess Oil

Pimples are caused by clogged pores that get infected with accumulated bacteria called *P. acnes*. Pus builds up and you have the dreaded whitehead. The best way to tackle bacteria is with a cleanser containing **benzoyl peroxide**. This kills *P. acnes* and is also anti-inflammatory, so it helps to reduce redness. Ten percent benzoyl peroxide cream (in addition to a benzoyl peroxide–based cleanser) can mop up excess oil quite effectively.

If you are prone to both pimples and blackheads, try alternating cleansers every other day: one with salicylic acid and one with benzoyl peroxide.

Step Three: Increase Cell Turnover

One of the best antiaging creams also happens to be one of the most effective ways to treat acne by causing more efficient cell turnover, which helps pores unclog naturally. I'm talking about tretinoin. **Tretinoin** is a prescription medication, but most doctors will prescribe it for problematic adult acne. **Adapalene** (also known as **Differin**) is another prescription cream that works similarly to tretinoin, but it can also come premixed with benzoyl peroxide under the trade name **Epiduo**. If you don't want to get a prescription, then consider adding a retinol-based cream to your antiacne regimen. Just make sure it isn't too thick so it doesn't clog your pores.

Step Four: Know How to Manhandle Pimples

Because adult acne tends to be cystic, it's also important to know how to handle those big ones when they come in (right before you need to look fabulous, of course). I have a few tricks for this. Some of them you can do at home, and some you can do at the doctor's office.

* Ask your doctor to inject your pimple with **cortisone**. This is especially effective for those really deep, cystic pimples. It will speed up the healing—the pimple should disappear within two to three days.

* Try the **Tanda Zap**. This is a device you use at home that treats pimples with blue light to kill bacteria and warmth to increase blood supply, as well as vibration to clear pores. This handy device can zap a pimple within twenty-four hours if you start using it when the pimple first appears. It retails for just $39.99, which I think is a good deal for a tool you can use over and over again.

* A spot of **toothpaste** (use only the kind that is all white in color) can dry out a pimple within a few hours. Dab it on before you go to bed, and wake up with a zit that is just a shadow of its former self.

* One simple method for reducing the inflammation of a pimple is to apply a **Band-Aid** over it. Studies show that a covered wound heals better than one that is open to the air. Therefore, I've found that covering a pimple with a Band-Aid, even if just overnight, can reduce the redness and inflammation, causing it to heal and disappear faster. This trick can be combined with any of the treatments above for maximal effect.

* Oral **zinc supplements** can be helpful for some people with acne, due to zinc's anti-inflammatory effect. One study showed that taking 30 mg of **zinc** per day was effective in reducing acne, although it was less effective than the antibiotic minocycline.[8] There are several commercially available formulations of zinc made specifically for acne. Most of these contain a slightly higher dose of 50 mg per day. Studies also show that combining zinc supplements with **oral antibiotics** may aid in preventing antibiotic resistance.[9]

* Don't throw away that **banana peel**! Rub it on your face instead. Cut off a small piece, about one inch square, and rub the inside of the peel onto areas where you have acne until the inside of the peel turns brown. Allow the banana residue to dry on your face and leave it on for thirty minutes while you do something else. Wash it off with warm water and repeat two or three times per day. (Save the peel in an airtight bag in the refrigerator.) The reason this helps with acne is that banana peels contain fatty acids and antioxidants that soothe skin. For this reason, banana peels are also good for other skin issues like eczema and psoriasis. Just be sure to consult with your dermatologist if you want to try this for a more serious skin disorder.

Although banana peels can do nice things for your skin, I do recommend a visit to a dermatologist if you have severe acne, such as full-face acne with cystic areas. The humble banana can do only so much.

If the above topical treatments don't improve your acne, then you probably need a visit to the dermatologist. The combination of prescribed oral antibiotics (like doxycycline) with benzoyl peroxide or a retinoid like tretinoin (see Step Three) may be needed to effectively attack chronic adult acne. Not only does doxycycline kill *P. acnes*, but it also acts as a general anti-inflammatory to reduce the

Caution!

If oral antibiotics combined with the above treatments don't work, then the next step would be to consider hormone manipulation (such as with birth control pills) or **isotretinoin** (otherwise known as **Accutane**). Isotretinoin is usually considered the treatment of last resort for acne. Although it is extremely effective in clearing even the worst cystic acne, there are potential side effects. It's also extremely important not to get pregnant if you are on isotretinoin, due to the potential risk of birth defects.

appearance of new lesions. It doesn't work immediately, but many people find their acne lesions becoming less and less common after a month or two of treatment.

AGE SPOTS, SUN SPOTS, LIVER SPOTS, AND MELASMA

Besides wrinkles and fine lines and the indignity of adult acne, the biggest sign of aging on the face is age spots, sometimes called sun spots or liver spots. A variation of this is a condition called melasma, in which dark patches develop on the face, usually related to sun exposure.

Sun spots are darkened spots on the face. They can also appear on the chest, arms, hands, or anywhere else you get regular sun exposure. They have a variety of appearances, from light to dark, flat to elevated, freckle-sized to large. Sometimes many spots can clump together, making the appearance of a large blotch of pigment. These spots also have a variety of names, including freckles, age spots, liver spots (although they have nothing to do with the liver—they are called this because they can be liver colored), and solar lentigines. In most cases, sun spots are the result of UV radiation, which causes the melanocytes in your skin to produce melanin in an attempt to protect the skin from the radiation. In general, these spots do not disappear spontaneously. The only way to get rid of them is to do something to them.

Melasma is a slightly different but similar problem. It's caused by hereditary factors and hormones (it can occur during pregnancy) as well as sun exposure. Instead of cute little freckles or charming moles, melasma involves large, dark patches on the face that occur on sun-exposed areas like the cheeks and forehead. The longer you have a melasma patch without treating it, the harder it is to fade. New spots can fade quickly with over-the-counter creams (I discuss these just a little bit later in the chapter), but older spots are more stubborn and may require medical treatment.

Here are some general therapies that can make a real difference in the appearance of age spots, sun spots, liver spots, and melasma.

Intense Pulsed Light Therapy (IPL): The best treatment for age spots, and an ✸ **AGE FIX FAVORITE** , is a procedure called intense pulsed light therapy (IPL). This is also sometimes called a **FotoFacial**. IPL treatments target dark spots and destroy them with pulsed light, which causes the spots to turn slightly darker and eventually slough off. IPL treatments are generally painless and require no downtime or recovery. They can be used to treat sun spots on all parts of the body, including the face, chest, and hands.

This procedure is performed across the country in plastic surgery and dermatology offices. It typically costs several hundred dollars per treatment, and four to six treatments are usually required for optimal results.

Chemical peels can also be very effective at removing sun spots. I prefer IPL treatments over chemical peels, however, since the lighter, lunchtime chemical peels are usually not aggressive enough to remove sun spots. Most of the time, more aggressive peels are needed, and these come with significant peeling and downtime. Most of my patients would rather spend a little more to have a FotoFacial and avoid having to take the time to peel.

For melasma, especially stubborn patches, the best medical treatment is to combine creams (see the next section) with IPL and chemical peels and/or laser treatments. Chemical peels will treat only superficial melasma unless the peel is quite intense. IPL and laser treatments are better at treating melasma spots that have deeper pigment, because these treatments pass through the upper layers of the skin.

Fountain of Youth

Even better than treating sun spots is preventing them. This is where **sunblock** comes in. Sun spots arise from not only the sun damage that you are currently subjecting your skin to, but also the sun damage from years and years ago. Start early, and teach your kids to protect their skin, too. Apply sunblock to your children so they won't have to deal with premature aging like many of us are having to do. For more information on sunblock, check the next chapter.

Ultimate 3-in-1 Antiaging Face Cream: There is a topical treatment for pigment issues that you can use at home. I consider it one of my **AGE FIX FAVORITES** because it is quite powerful: the Ultimate 3-in-1 Antiaging Face Cream. This isn't a specific product you can buy, but a method of combining three different products in a way that is very effective. This is my favorite way to treat pigmentation on the face and is, in my opinion, probably the best available cream combination for treating melasma.

This special concoction combines two of the most effective antiaging creams: **tretinoin**, the only scientifically proven cream to tighten skin, reduce fine lines, and even reverse early precancerous skin lesions; and **4% (or more) hydroquinone**, the most powerful pigment-reducing cream, available in the prescription strength of 4%. Combining these two creams can result in better penetration and the maximal effectiveness in reducing age spots and sun damage.

The third component of this combination is a steroid to reduce the common skin reaction to tretinoin: redness, itching, and flaking. I recommend a very small amount of **hydrocortisone cream 0.5%.** This is typically not enough to create the severe thinning that can occur with higher-potency steroid creams.

Because you cannot buy this combination of creams—they are prescription strength and not made by any manufacturers—you will need to ask your plastic surgeon or dermatologist to have it made by their compound pharmacy.

Apply it every other night at first, increasing to every night as tolerated. Once your skin looks better, decrease or discontinue its use, since it's not a good idea to apply the hydrocortisone or hydroquinone to your skin indefinitely. Make sure to consult with a board-certified dermatologist or plastic surgeon prior to starting this treatment, to confirm that it is right for you and your skin issues.

Beauty Secret

I also recommend the **Obagi Nu-Derm** skin-care line, and the newer **ZO Medical** skin-care line. These prescription-strength skin-care lines, which are two of my favorite of all the medical skin-care regimens, are based on tretinoin and 4% hydroquinone. Both are extremely potent and effective in reducing pigmentary issues like melasma and sun spots. I don't think there are more effective lines of skin-care products available to reduce pigment, improve fine lines, and tighten the skin. ZO also has a nonhydroquinone and nontretinoin regimen that is recommended for those who are sensitive to these ingredients. ZO Medical is the highest-selling skin-care line in my practice in Michigan.

   Depending on where you live, you may not have access to a plastic surgeon or dermatologist. If this is the case, head over to your local drugstore and check out L'Oréal's **Youth Code Dark Spot Corrector**. It contains niacinamide, a gradual age-spot reducer. Although it will probably take longer to fade your sun spots when compared to Obagi or ZO products, it costs less than $30 and is pretty mild on the skin.

Licorice Root: Licorice root is an all-natural product that some skin-lightening creams contain, or you can use the extract itself. Purchase **licorice root extract drops** in your local health-food store or online, and apply the liquid with a cotton swab directly to brown spots every morning and every evening. You should see fading in about two months.

DIY Sunspot-Lightening Mask: You can make this mask at home from ingredients you probably already have in your kitchen. Combine 1 tablespoon each of **soy milk,** **honey,** and **lemon juice** in a small bowl. Apply to your face, and let it sit for twenty to thirty minutes. Wash it off with warm water. Repeat two to three times per week, and you should notice sun spots fading after eight to ten weeks. All for just pennies! This works because the citric acid in lemon juice is a natural skin lightener, soy milk has enzymes that can inhibit the production of melanin in the skin (and is also full of vitamins A and E, which are both good for aging skin), and honey is what I call the jack-of-all-trades for at-home skin care. It has natural antibacterial properties, so it can help reduce acne; it also soothes irritated skin, moisturizes dry skin, and tightens the skin. It's a great ingredient to add to most at-home skin-care regimens.

Beauty Secret

Makeup can also help to hide age spots pretty effectively. Find a yellow-based concealer that is two shades lighter than your normal skin color. Thicker concealers like Dermablend usually work well.

* Apply the concealer with your finger or a brush.

* Pat your foundation over the areas. Be careful if you rub the foundation, as it can cause the concealer to smudge.

* Apply powder over the foundation to set it.

Now that you have some good, targeted information on how to tackle the most pressing aging issues on the part of you that faces the world every day, let's get into prevention and routine maintenance of your skin. In the next chapter, I'll take you through a routine you can customize for your own needs, lifestyle, and budget.

4 THE AGE-FIX ROUTINE

So far, we've talked about how skin ages and some of the things you can do to treat specific aging features on your skin. However, the real foundation of ways to combat aging is in your daily routine. How you treat your skin every morning and every evening will affect your skin quality and youthfulness in a way that provides a solid base for the wrinkle treatments, fine line attacks, and even procedures like Botox.

Skin care is confusing. Department stores are filled with so many brands and so many products that it can make even the most educated, savvy consumer feel a little bit bewildered. In fact, one report estimated that in 2013, over $55 billion was spent on cosmetics, much of this on products to look younger.[10] I once had a patient ask me for advice on which products were best for her skin. I requested that she bring her products with her to her next appointment so we could determine together which ones to use and which ones to discard. A week later, she carted in a huge garbage bag filled with half-empty bottles and tubes of lotions, potions, and cleansers! Unfortunately, I don't think she's alone. Most women have dozens of partially used beauty products filling their bathroom cabinets, shelves, and drawers. This chapter is going to tell you what to do with them. Most of them are unnecessary and should go in the garbage (or recycle bin). A handful can really make your skin look better.

This chapter will help you separate the necessary products from the products that are simply a waste of your money. I'll also help you establish that all-important routine so you can stop contributing to aging and start reversing the aging process today. In fact, I like to think of it as an Age-Fix routine, rather than merely a skin-care routine, because that's exactly what we are doing—optimizing your skin quality specifically so you look as ageless as possible.

THE AGE-FIX SCHEDULE

Your basic Age-Fix routine really is relatively simple. All it takes is three steps: cleansing, treating, and protecting, each practiced twice per day. These three simple steps (with the right products for you) can go a very long way toward keeping you looking younger longer. The younger you are when you start, the better this Age-Fix routine will preserve the good skin you've already got, but it's never too late to turn back the clock. You can start at any age and look younger almost immediately. Let's start today! More specifically, here's what you will be doing:

EVERY MORNING:

1. You will cleanse your skin with a cleanser that is appropriate for your skin type.

2. You will treat your skin with the appropriate serum.

3. Finally, you will protect your skin with moisturizer and sunscreen.

EVERY EVENING:

1. You will cleanse your skin, removing makeup with a product we will tailor to your skin type. You will also cleanse away the day's debris, oil, and pollution. In the evening a few times a week we will also include exfoliation, which is a preparatory step for treatment.

2. You will treat your skin with the appropriate serum, which is particularly essential before sleep.

3. Finally, you will protect your skin, but this time it won't be with sunscreen. It will be with the night cream that is best for you.

Let's look at each part separately so you can pick out some products.

CLEANSING

Cleansing is the foundation for effective skin care, because clean skin can maintain itself with the least interference, and it can best absorb products that combat aging. Cleansing is particularly important at night. Like the rest of the body, skin restores itself at night.

Having its pores clogged with oil and makeup and its crevices filled with dust, grime, germs, and pollution can prevent this from happening, in addition to increasing the risk of breakouts.

Cleansing your skin in both the morning and the evening will get rid of external dirt and internally produced oil that can give skin a dull look. Cleansing, and particularly exfoliating, also helps to sweep away that very top layer of dead skin, revealing fresher, younger-looking skin.

However, many women cleanse their skin incorrectly, either not cleaning it thoroughly enough or cleaning it too harshly. Cleansing should leave your face feeling clean and comfortably tight. It should never make your face red or sting, or cause the skin to feel dry and look flaky.

Apply cleanser in a circular motion using clean hands. The circular motion gently massages your face and stimulates blood flow and oxygenation of the skin. Rinse with warm water, and then pat dry with a clean towel.

How do you know what kind of cleanser to use? Before you can determine this, you must first know what your skin type is.

Caution!

Different skin types require different types of cleanser, but there is one common cleanser nobody should ever use: common bar soap. Soap often contains a drying surfactant called sodium lauryl sulfate, which can leave a film on your skin that feels uncomfortable, strip it of essential oils, and deplete moisture. Even worse, drying your skin can increase the appearance of wrinkles.

Find Your Skin Type

You may already know what kind of skin you have—oily, dry, combination. Maybe you know how your skin used to be as a teenager or a young adult, but you aren't sure what's happening lately. Or maybe you have no idea. You just wash your face and move on with your life.

Knowing your skin type is actually quite useful, because it allows you to tailor products to your exact skin type, which means you will get better results from the products you use. Skin type can change as you age, too. A teenager with oily skin can grow into a woman with dry skin, and a young woman with normal skin can develop oily or dry or especially combination skin as she gets older. To find what your skin type is today, here's a simple test:

1. Wash your face with a gentle facial cleanser, rinse, and pat dry with a soft towel.

2. Wait sixty minutes.

3. Blot your face with a tissue. Look at your skin and the tissue.

   Dry skin: If your skin is dry, then sixty minutes after washing, it will look a bit flaky and feel tight. No oil will be on the tissue.

   Sensitive skin: If you have sensitive skin, you may notice redness, itching, or even a rash after cleansing.

   Normal skin: If you have normal skin, then your skin will feel slightly tight but comfortable without flaking and without oil on the tissue.

   Oily skin: If you have oily skin, there will be oil on the tissue from most or all of the areas of your face.

   Combination skin: If you have combination skin, you could have a combination of oil in areas like the T-zone, flaky skin in areas like the cheeks, and normal skin in areas like the chin.

Cleanser Matchup

The first thing to do, now that you know your skin type, is to find the best cleanser for you. There are a slew of them out there, but don't just grab the first one you see (or the one you've been using since you were seventeen). Cleansers should leave your face feeling clean and tight but not too tight, never greasy but also never red, stinging, dry, flaky, or irritated. Some cleansers come with gentle exfoliating particles. Other cleansers aren't even meant to be washed off with water, and should be gently wiped off with a tissue.

Is your cleanser still right for you? Maybe not. Here are the best cleanser types for your skin. You'll notice I've included some subcategories, such as "very dry" and "slightly dry," as well as conflating some categories, like "normal to oily." This allows you to customize further. Try a few different things before settling on the one that makes your skin look and feel fantastic after using it. Also keep in mind that the cleanser that works for you this year might not work so well a few years from now. Always pay attention to how your skin reacts to your Age-Fix routine, and always be willing to try new things when something isn't working as well anymore.

* **For very dry, very sensitive skin:** Use a surfactant-free cleanser that doesn't require rinsing. Just the act of rinsing the skin with tap water can worsen the driest, most sensitive skin. If that sounds like you, there are a handful of "no-rinse" cleansers that are very mild, preserve as much moisture as possible, and don't require you to rinse them off. **Pond's Cold Cream Cleanser** is a very affordable old standby that many people still use to clean the skin while still maintaining hydration. My favorite in this category is **Avène Extremely Gentle Cleansing Lotion**. It's a little pricier but is devoid of fragrances and parabens. Add a spray of thermal spring water (such as **Avène Thermal Spring Water spray**) after you've wiped it off with a tissue for best results.

* **For slightly sensitive, slightly dry skin:** Try a creamy cleanser that will leave your skin feeling slightly moisturized. An inexpensive choice is **CeraVe Hydrating Cleanser**, with ceramides and hyaluronic acid to moisturize the skin. **Philosophy Purity Made Simple Cleanser** costs more but is fragrance free and contains natural oils that can leave your skin feeling lightly moisturized. Both of these should be gently rinsed off with tap water.

* **For normal to oily skin:** Try a foaming cleanser. This will clean skin more aggressively and is particularly effective at removing makeup. However, because of the more aggressive cleansing, foaming cleansers can be drying and irritating to sensitive skin. An inexpensive choice is **Neutrogena Fresh Foaming Cleanser**. A splurge is **Epionce Gentle Foaming Cleanser**, which retains the natural oils of the skin better than most foaming cleansers.

Do You Need Toner?

Toners were popular back when most cleansers left an oily residue behind. They were astringents that made the skin feel cool and clean, but they were also harsh, stripping skin of its natural oils, and could cause excessive drying. Rubbing alcohol feels cool on the skin, too, but that doesn't mean you should rub it all over your face!

As long as your cleanser doesn't leave behind a palpable residue, you probably don't need toner. If you have very dry skin, eczema, or rosacea, you should not use toner. However, if you have very oily skin, you can use toner up to twice a day, which can help decrease oiliness and shine. In my office we recommend **Cebatrol Oil Control Pads** by ZO Medical Products.

Under the right circumstances and with the right product, toners can reduce inflammation and soothe skin. For nonoily skin, I recommend alcohol-free toners that specifically act to balance skin pH, such as **NARS Multi-Action Hydrating Toner**.

All About Exfoliation

Exfoliation is an important and often overlooked way to expose younger skin and even regenerate skin cells. It can be part of cleansing, or it can be separate from cleansing. A large portion of the upper layers of our skin is composed of dead or dying skin cells. These dead skin cells can cause a flat or dull look to our skin. Exfoliating will help remove the upper layers of dead skin and speed up cellular turnover, which starts to slow down in the twenties and thirties.

Basically, exfoliation causes the cells to send signals to produce new skin cells. It also stimulates the production of new collagen fibers, replacing the damaged, irregular, and aged collagen fibers. Exfoliation can reverse the thinning of the collagen in the dermis that occurs with aging, and it also enhances the work of treatment creams and serums. This is why I prefer evening for exfoliation. Removing the top layers of dead skin will make it easier for your night cream to penetrate into the deeper layers of skin. For best results, always exfoliate after you cleanse, so you are exfoliating a fresh, clean face.

There are really three ways to exfoliate, and you may find that one or two of these work for you but not all three. Or you may find (especially if you have very sensitive skin) that you don't need to exfoliate much at all. Here are the types and levels:

1. **Physically:** Some cleansers or other topical products contain tiny microbeads meant to gently abrade the top layers of skin. This is considered to be the gentlest kind of exfoliation. However, I really don't think these beads do much of anything, and one study even suggests that these beads can be hazardous to the environment.[11] For these reasons, I recommend you steer clear of cleansers with microbeads. Instead, two better ways to physically exfoliate your skin are to use a handheld cleansing and exfoliating device (like the Clarisonic) or to use a gritty skin polisher. Currently, my favorite physical exfoliating polish is the **ZO Skin Health Offects Exfoliating Polish**. It combines ultrafine magnesium crystals with antioxidants for an effective, gentle exfoliation. Another great option, **Epicuren Micro-Derm Ultra-Refining Scrub**, contains ecofriendly bamboo microcrystals that can gently exfoliate your skin.

2. **Chemically:** Cleansers or other topical products can contain alpha- or beta-hydroxy acids, which remove the top layers of skin through chemical action. I'll talk more about these in the treatment section, but this is a more aggressive exfoliation that can unveil younger skin but may be too harsh for very sensitive skin.

3. **Enzymatically:** Cleansers or other topical products can contain botanical extracts to exfoliate the skin through their enzymatic action. I'll also talk more about these in the treatment section, but this kind of exfoliation can range from aggressive to gentle, depending on the product.

Exfoliation is effective, but you can also overdo it. If you have sensitive skin, exfoliate one or two times per week at most. If you have normal skin, you can exfoliate every other day. If your skin gets red and irritated, that's a sign that you are exfoliating too often. Slow it down and find a level of exfoliation that doesn't irritate you but still keeps your skin looking fresh and smooth.

Caution!

Do not exfoliate your eyelids or the skin directly beneath your eye (the lower lid area). This skin is typically too sensitive to tolerate the harshness of exfoliation, and you also don't want to risk getting any exfoliating product in your eyes.

DIY BAKING SODA CLEANSER/EXFOLIATOR

I'm not a huge fan of making your own cleanser, since cleansers are, in general, pretty inexpensive to purchase and there really aren't a lot of benefits to DIY cleansers, compared to some of the other DIY recipes in this book. Unless you really want to save money and be as natural as possible with what you put on your skin, it's probably best to just buy a good, inexpensive cleanser like **Neutrogena Fresh Foaming Cleanser** if you can't afford a nicer, pricier one, like the **Clinique Rinse-Off Foaming Cleanser**.

However, I do like this one, because baking soda is a natural exfoliator and can even have a subtle, gentle lightening effect. Your skin will feel clean and fresh after you use this. Make this fresh each time you want to use it, and use the whole thing—it does not keep well due to the milk.

1 tablespoon baking soda

½ teaspoon honey

¼ cup reduced-fat milk

1. Gently warm the milk on the stove or briefly in the microwave, just until it starts to steam, but not so long that it bubbles or scalds. Watch it closely!

2. Stir all the ingredients together in a bowl.

3. Rinse your face with warm water, put the cleanser on a washcloth, and gently clean your skin with it. Rinse off with warm water.

TREATMENT

Clean, exfoliated skin is prepared for treatment, and there are many excellent ways to treat your skin, depending on what your issues are. Check out these various treatments and what they do so you can choose the ones that will tackle the specific issues you have now.

Retinoids

No matter your issue, unless your skin is very sensitive, retinoids just may be your new best friend. Retinoids are really just various types of vitamin A, which is the vitamin contained (in the form of beta-carotene) in orange fruits and vegetables like carrots, pumpkins, peaches, and apricots. Sounds pretty ho-hum, right? Wrong! If I could choose one type of topical treatment for the skin, no question it would be a retinoid. Retinoids do it all. They exfoliate the skin, gradually lighten dark spots, act as anti-inflammatory agents, tighten the skin, reduce fine lines, and even increase the thickness of the skin, which is especially important for the thin skin of the eyelids (more on that later). Retinoids can effectively treat both pimples and wrinkles, and they are one of the most effective products for either issue—and an Age-Fix lifesaver if you suffer from both at the same time, as so many perimenopausal women do. Even more impressive, some studies have shown that prescription-strength retinoids can actually reverse early pre-skin-cancer changes in the skin and actual pre-skin-cancer lesions like actinic keratoses.[12] Impressive, right?

There are two types of retinoids: prescription-strength tretinoin and the milder, over-the-counter retinol. These products are best applied at bedtime, allowing them six to eight hours to penetrate and affect the skin while you sleep.

RETIN-A

Retin-A is the brand name for tretinoin, and with daily use you may see acne clearing up within two weeks, and wrinkles smoothing and skin tightening within a month or two. It comes in three prescription strengths: 0.1%, 0.05%, and 0.025%. Use a pea-sized amount on your skin every other night to every night, as directed by your doctor. Apply it only at night, because light will deactivate it. You may develop irritation of the skin, dryness, flaking, or a dermatitis within a few days of starting tretinoin. It is also possible that you will experience an initial, temporary period of increased acne. These symptoms typically resolve with continued use, but if you develop these types of symptoms, consult with your doctor. He or she may recommend that you decrease the frequency of use until your skin gets used to it, or prescribe a lesser strength.

The first time I tried Retin-A, I was in medical school. My family physician, who didn't have much experience in prescribing it, started my wife and me on 0.1% every night and instructed us to slather it on. Three days later, both our faces were beet-red, swollen, painful, and peeling. Our faces felt as if they were on fire, and we looked like a pair of lobsters.

Unless you have the skin of an elephant, it may be best to ask your doctor to start you on a lower strength of tretinoin until you know your skin can tolerate it. This can be frustrating, because the higher the strength of tretinoin, the sooner you will see the positive effects. Slowing down use because of irritation can also slow down results, but be patient and stick with it! Let your skin adjust. You will see results from this **AGE FIX FAVORITE**. Tretinoin is quite effective as long as you stick with the program. Although some patients just can't tolerate tretinoin, most of us can as long as we allow our skin to gradually get used to it.

There are also some other versions of tretinoin, or Retin-A. **Retin-A Micro** contains the same amount of the active ingredient but is a less irritating formulation, and **Renova** (or its similar competitor, **ReFissa**) is a more moisturizing form of Retin-A. While your prescription medication insurance may cover generic tretinoin or Retin-A Micro to treat acne, it never covers Renova or ReFissa. These two are considered cosmetic products for the sole purpose of reversing aging.

Caution!

Tretinoin can sensitize your skin to sunlight, making you more prone to burning and the aging effects of the sun. If you are using tretinoin, be sure to stay out of the sun, or wear a strong sunblock with a high SPF (I'll talk more about sunblock in the "Protection" section of this chapter). Tretinoin may be contraindicated for people with very dark skin and should definitely not be used if you are pregnant or nursing. Also, avoid applying tretinoin directly to your sensitive eyelid skin, as it may be too strong. Consult with your doctor about whether tretinoin is right for you.

RETINOL

Retinol is a weaker, over-the-counter form of retinoid that is not as fast acting as tretinoin but may be more appropriate for those who find prescription-strength tretinoin to be too strong. Studies have shown that although retinol is not as potent as tretinoin, it can have similar antiaging effects.

Most major skin-care manufacturers with antiaging lines carry retinol-based products. They don't typically give you an exact percentage of retinol in their product, so unfortunately the best way to determine which retinol cream is best for you is through trial and error. Two of my favorites are **SkinCeuticals Retinol 1.0** and **Revision Retinol Facial Repair.** For a less expensive option, you can check out the retinol-based serums and creams at your local drugstore, such as **Neutrogena's Rapid Wrinkle Repair** and **RoC Retinol Correxion.**

DIY APRICOT FACE MASK

Retinoids are an active form of vitamin A, and apricots are chock-full of vitamin A, which is why many face products contain apricot ingredients. You can take advantage of this by creating your own face mask full of vitamin A. Your face will feel softer, smoother, and more moisturized afterward, like a baby's butt! It will also smell great. The smell of this mask reminds me of the high-end skin-care line called **Epicuren.** They have a number of products that smell like apricots.

Warning: This mask can be a bit messy, especially if you apply it yourself. If you have another person apply it with an inexpensive makeup brush, it may go on better (and feel more like a spa experience). Also, rinse this off in your kitchen sink, as tiny pieces of apricot could clog your bathroom drain.

½ cup dried apricots

½ cup warm water

1 tablespoon raw honey

Blend all the ingredients in a blender or Magic Bullet until the mixture is pureed and smooth. Spread the mask on your face and let it sit for twenty minutes. Discard any extra. Rinse your face with warm water and apply a facial moisturizer.

ANTIOXIDANTS

Antioxidants are in many of the foods we eat, especially colorful fruits and vegetables. They include things like vitamin C, vitamin E, and even the vitamin A that makes up retinoids. They also include other antioxidants such as coenzyme Q10 and manganese. What makes a substance an antioxidant is its ability to repair and prevent damage from free radicals in the body by neutralizing them.

I like antioxidants for antiaging used both internally (in the diet and in supplements) and externally, on the skin. They fight aging, sagging, wrinkles, and even skin cancer. They provide a protective effect, and while they don't reverse previous damage, they can do a lot to prevent future damage.

I recommend using an antioxidant cream in the morning so it can protect your skin during the day. Ingredients in many skin-care products that signify antioxidant content include:

* Vitamin C

* Vitamin E

* Green tea

* Black tea

* Coenzyme Q10

* Pomegranate

* Soy

Vitamin C is one of the most common and effective antioxidant ingredients in skin-care products, and it is often included in serums. Look for at least 10% L-ascorbic acid in the ingredients if you want the vitamin C to have an effect. Also, vitamin C is relatively unstable and must be packed correctly or it will degrade. A vitamin C product should always be in a dark container, because light will oxidize it, causing it to lose effectiveness. If your vitamin C serum turns dark yellow or brown, throw it away. It has oxidized. ZO Medical Products has a great moisturizing 10% vitamin C serum called **C-Bright**.

Vitamin C's best friend and partner is vitamin E. A study in the *Journal of the American Academy of Dermatology* found that the effects of topical vitamin C are enhanced when combined with vitamin E, another potent antioxidant.[13] Combining antioxidants can actually be synergistic! SkinCeuticals has a fantastic combo product called **CE Ferulic**, an ✳ AGE FIX FAVORITE with 15% L-ascorbic acid and 1% alpha-tocopherol, a type of vitamin E. Its effects can last seventy-two hours after the application.

DIY Pineapple Scrub

Vitamin C treatments are easy to make at home with fresh fruit. One of the most potent sources is pineapple, which works hard for you in this great, gritty scrub that uses cornmeal as an exfoliator. The exfoliation effect will help the vitamin C to penetrate more effectively, making your skin feel smooth and rejuvenated. Repeat twice per week, as long as this treatment doesn't irritate your skin. (Discontinue if you notice any redness or irritation. This treatment should feel good, but it may not agree with all skin types.)

½ cup cubed or chopped pineapple, preferably fresh	**Puree the pineapple with the water. Add the cornmeal and blend just until combined. Gently apply the scrub to your face and massage. After a few minutes, wash off with warm water. Store any extra in an airtight container in the refrigerator. It should last for two to three days.**
¼ cup warm water	
3 tablespoons cornmeal	

ALPHA-HYDROXY ACIDS (AHAs)

Alpha-hydroxy acids (AHAs) include three kinds of acids that naturally occur in common foods: fruit acids, glycolic acids, and lactic acids. These light acids exfoliate the skin, removing the upper layer of dead skin cells and exposing the younger, smoother layer underneath. This stimulates new cell growth.

The most effective of the AHAs is glycolic acid, which comes from sugarcane. The small size of the glycolic acid particles allows for better penetration into the skin. However, glycolic acid is also the most likely to cause irritation, so if you have sensitive skin, glycolic acid may not be the best choice for you.

Lactic acid comes from milk and acts as a good moisturizer as well as a gentle exfoliator. Women in ancient Egypt, including (according to legend) Cleopatra, used to bathe in milk for its beautifying effects. Somehow, they knew about the antiaging properties of lactic acid.

Fruit acids include citric acid from citrus fruits.

AHAs can be used as stand-alone peels or serums, or incorporated into exfoliating cleansers. Look for products with 7% or higher content of AHA for the best results. (Doctors often prescribe AHAs in a strength of 20–30%.) Everyone's skin has a different tolerance for AHAs. Some people tolerate them well and benefit from a stronger percentage in order to see results. Ideally, pick a strength that gives some initial flaking of the skin that resolves quickly and doesn't cause extended redness or irritation.

Many over-the-counter products do not list their AHA percentages, and this is probably on purpose, because many of them don't contain enough to make a difference. However, there are some I like because I've seen noticeable effects with their use. La Roche-Posay has a nice AHA serum called **Effaclar Pore Refining Anti-Wrinkle Serum** that boasts 7.5% AHA-glycolic complex.

Insider Tip

I find that AHAs have the best results when combined with tretinoin. AHAs work on the surface and tretinoin works deep in the skin for a potent inside-outside combination. Make sure to seek a plastic surgeon's or dermatologist's advice when combining these two, since your skin may find the duo too aggressive.

Because AHA Ingredients Are So Common in Foods, It's Easy to Make Effective DIY Products at Home.

DIY AHA Mask

This mask uses fruit acids from the orange juice and lemon juice and lactic acid from the yogurt. It also contains a nice dose of vitamin C.

3 tablespoons orange juice

2 tablespoons lemon juice

¾ cup plain (unsweetened, unflavored) yogurt

Mix these ingredients together with a fork until combined and apply to your face. Let the mixture sit for twenty minutes, or until dry. Rinse it off with warm water. Your skin will feel softer and smoother afterward.

Growth Factors

Growth factors are a little more complex, but they can have a dramatic effect on your skin. They are chemical messengers that can signal the skin cells to increase the production of new collagen. Growth factors have been effectively used for many years in wound healing, and they now have become an essential ingredient in the antiaging creams and serums of many skin-care products. They can be a good replacement for retinoids if your skin cannot tolerate those, because they cause much less irritation, flaking, and drying. If I had to choose between a retinol-based cream and a growth factor–based cream, I'd go with the retinol, since the science to support its antiaging effects on the skin is clearer and retinols are, in general, less expensive. However, if these just don't work for you, consider growth factors.

Neocutis and SkinMedica are two examples of skin-care companies that reportedly use growth factors in their products. I've had many, many patients who swear by **SkinMedica's TNS Essential Serum** as an integral part of their skin-care regimen. I first encountered this product many years ago but was immediately turned off by its strong smell. Since then, the scent has been greatly improved, and for most it's no longer an issue.

If you'd like to see how growth factors may improve your skin, then SkinMedica's TNS Essential Serum or **TNS Recovery Complex** are considered by many dermatologists and plastic surgeons to be the gold standard.

Neocutis's products aren't as talked about as SkinMedica's. Still, its line of Bio-Restorative skin creams is worth a look, especially its **Bio-Restorative Serum**. Both SkinMedica and Neocutis products are sold in doctors' offices. My main issue with growth factor–based skin products is the price. They can cost over $200 for as little as one ounce of product! It's like liquid gold! Therefore, again, I recommend that you try retinoids first.

PEPTIDES

Peptides are another common antiaging ingredient in skin-care products. They come in three forms, each with its own specific benefits.

The first type of peptide improves the skin by prompting the cells to increase collagen production. As the collagen in our skin degrades with age, it releases small proteins. These proteins signal the skin to create new collagen to take the place of the degraded collagen. Peptides, such as Matrixyl, Dermaxyl, and oligopeptides, are small chains of proteins that can potentially do this as well, signaling the dermis to create more collagen and rejuvenate aged skin.[14] Peptide-based products are, in general, less expensive than growth factor–based products. You can find these types of collagen-enhancing peptides in the **Oil of Olay Regenerist** line and **StriVectin's Advanced Intensive Concentrate for Wrinkles and Stretch Marks**. Both can be found in your local drugstore or online.

The second type of peptide acts as a carrier for copper, allowing the combination to penetrate the skin and affect its structure. Copper has been used for decades to improve wound healing and has been incorporated into skin-care products since 1997. Copper peptides are believed to have many beneficial effects on aging skin, including increasing the production of hyaluronic acid (a moisturizing component of the skin) and collagen, and acting as an antioxidant. If you'd like to see how copper peptides improve your skin, check out the **Progressive Nourishing Lotion** or **Crème de la Copper** by NEOVA. These can be purchased online or through a physician's office.

The third type of peptide is collectively called neuropeptides. These include gamma-amino-butyric acid (GABA) and dimethylaminoethanol (DMAE). Studies show that GABA can act as a smooth muscle relaxer.[15] Smooth muscles are also called involuntary muscles, like the muscles of the GI tract, blood vessels, and uterus. If GABA can relax smooth muscles, can it also relax voluntary muscles like the ones that cause facial wrinkles? In other words, can it be like Botox in a cream form? Although rigorous scientific studies haven't proven that GABA in creams can penetrate the skin and relax the underlying facial muscles, it hasn't stopped some skin-care companies from claiming that it can and producing products that promise just that.

So what do I think of peptides? Should you look for creams and serums with peptides in them? Not necessarily. If you are a skin-care novice and want to maximize your dollars on your skin-care products, then hold off on buying peptide-based products. The science to support their benefits isn't very strong, and there are other, proven, less expensive ways to make your skin look better. However, if you are a seasoned veteran of skin-care products or a skin-care enthusiast, and you want to try something different, peptide-based creams and serums may be worth a try. Just don't believe *all* the hype.

SKIN LIGHTENERS

If you have dark spots, age spots, freckles, or melasma (all of which I discussed in the last chapter), you may want to try a skin-lightening treatment for the treatment step of your Age-Fix routine. You have a few options:

Hydroquinone: The gold standard for skin lightening is an ingredient called hydroquinone. This is a chemical compound that inhibits tyrosinase, a key enzyme essential in producing melanin (the pigment in the skin). The standard strength for hydroquinone in an over-the-counter product is 2%. Prescription strength is 4%. Hydroquinone works best when combined with retinoids and/or an AHA to get better penetration and quicker results (such as with the Ultimate 3-in-1 Antiaging Face Cream I told you about in chapter 3). For even better penetration, visit a plastic surgeon's or dermatologist's office and combine this with microdermabrasion. The microdermabrasion will gently exfoliate the skin and work with the hydroquinone to clear the dark spots faster.

Hands down, the best system for reducing pigmentation, in my humble opinion, is the **ZO Multi-Therapy Hydroquinone System**, my ✿ AGE FIX FAVORITE . While I do believe the 3-in-1 cream I recommended in the last chapter is the best single cream for pigmentation, it should not be used long-term. The ZO Medical system takes more steps but it is excellent for both short-term and longer-term use, and in that regard, I think it works even better for pigmentation than the 3-in-1 cream. This system combines 4% hydroquinone with tretinoin and AHAs for the most aggressive but well-tolerated skin-lightening regimen I've ever seen. I've witnessed amazing results with this system, but ideally you have to buy into the whole thing: cleanser, toner, exfoliator, lightener, blender, and sunscreen, which, taken together, appear to be synergistic with each other. If you have a lot of pigmentation problems that you need cleared up and cost isn't a barrier for you, then don't bother with the milder treatments. Go straight to ZO and see those spots lift within weeks. ZO Medical products can be purchased only through a physician's office.

> ## Caution!
>
> Hydroquinone is a very powerful topical agent, so improper use can be detrimental to your skin. In rare cases, people using hydroquinone can actually develop ochronosis, which causes a darkening of the skin. Because of this, hydroquinone has been banned in some European countries. However, this is a very rare complication.
>
> It's also important to avoid using prescription-strength hydroquinone on your skin for longer than six months at a time. Prolonged use can cause you to develop resistance to hydroquinone. Also, avoid using hydroquinone-based products if you are pregnant or nursing. That being said, don't be afraid to use hydroquinone to lighten your dark spots. I find that the benefits easily outweigh the risks, because hydroquinone is by far the most effective of all the products I've seen for lightening.

Kojic Acid: This is an alternate skin lightener that also works by inhibiting tyrosinase. It can be slightly more irritating than hydroquinone, but it is less expensive. Unlike hydroquinone, kojic acid doesn't come with the risk of ochronosis, but it also doesn't work quite as well. A recent study in the *Indian Journal of Dermatology* found that hydroquinone was more effective than kojic acid for the treatment of melasma. Because kojic acid is less effective than hydroquinone, it's best combined with an exfoliating agent for better penetration, such as an AHA or a retinoid. Otherwise, the results may be very mild and unsatisfactory.

Elure: Elure is a relatively new, nonhydroquinone, skin-lightening product marketed by Syneron, a prominent laser company. It has a patented natural enzyme formulation called Melanozyme, which can improve dark spots within twenty-eight days.

Niacinamide: Some over-the-counter skin-lightening products contain niacinamide, a very mild and gradual skin lightener. The good thing about niacinamide is that it's very safe, well tolerated, and inexpensive. The bad thing about it is that it works pretty slowly. L'Oréal has a nice, inexpensive skin lightener called **Youth Code Dark Spot Corrector**, which utilizes niacinamide. I mentioned this in the last chapter, so this is just a reminder.

PROTECTION

There is one thing you can do to protect your skin that far outweighs anything else. It is an essential practice for maintaining younger-looking skin, and it can even save your life. It's called sun protection.

I see you rolling your eyes at me! I know, people have been telling you to wear sunscreen ever since you were a sun-worshipping teenager, but you want your tan (or your vitamin D dose). Unfortunately, not everybody believes that sunscreen and sunblock are necessary unless, perhaps, you are at risk for burning, such as during a day at the beach. Many of these people claim that we need vitamin D from the sun and that sun is "natural" and that daily sunscreen use will lead to chronically low vitamin D levels. However, the aging effects of the sun are profound. Even if you don't burn, you will prematurely age if you get frequent sun exposure without protection. Is premature aging worth a temporary golden glow during the summer months? If you have darker skin, then the melanin in your skin can protect you from getting burned, but melanin will not protect you from getting wrinkles, pigmentary blotches, and skin cancer like melanoma. Sun protection is essential. My professional advice to you is to take a vitamin D supplement and embrace the sunscreen. Let's talk about how to use it.

Sunblock

I cannot overstate the importance of protecting young skin from the sun. It is always better to prevent skin damage than to treat it. This is especially important for children, so apply sunblock on your kids every day. Believe it or not, as much as 60 percent of the sun's damaging radiation penetrates the clouds, even on really cloudy days. You always need sunblock. *Always.* You need protection from both types of solar radiation that can damage and age your skin and cause cancer: UVA rays and UVB rays.

UVA rays: UVA rays cause aging, discoloration, and wrinkles, effects that can progress to skin cancer. These rays have a longer wavelength than UVB rays, so they penetrate deeper into the skin, at the molecular and cellular levels. Melanoma is caused by UVA rays, which react with the skin cells to produce free radicals. Free radicals caused by UVA rays can destroy DNA, sicken healthy cells, and damage collagen and elastin in your skin. This is what causes premature aging and sun damage. This damage can be even worse when combined with environmental free radicals like pollution and a poor diet.

A study conducted on twins by researchers from Case Western Reserve University showed an extra thirty hours a week of sun exposure made the subjects look 2 years older by age forty, and 3.5 years older by age seventy.[16] It can take ten years or more for the aging effects of the sun to surface on the skin, so your teenager's days at the pool without sunblock will affect her or him later, no matter what.

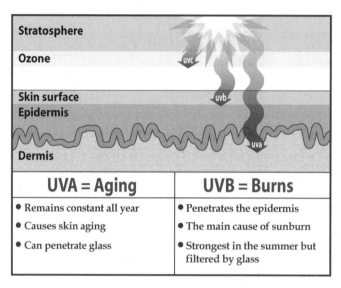

UVA vs. UVB RAYS

UVB rays: UVB rays are the ones that cause you to tan and also to burn. Long-term exposure to UVB rays is linked to basal cell and squamous cell carcinoma. UVB rays are most intense between 10 a.m. and 3 p.m., so try to limit your sun exposure at this time. Also keep in mind that the sun's rays are more intense near the equator and at higher altitudes. Also, being surrounded by snow, which reflects the sun's rays, can make it much easier for you to get burned. You may be surprised that higher altitudes make a difference, but they do. As a college student, I once took a ski trip to the Matterhorn in Switzerland. I'd never worn sunscreen while skiing before, but I slapped a little bit on my cheeks, just in case. When I finished skiing that day, my entire face was burned to a crisp, except for those two hand marks on each cheek and around my eyes where I wore my glasses. I looked like Free Willy. The other students made fun of me for weeks afterward, but I learned a valuable lesson. Even if it's cold, the sun's rays can still burn your skin. Apply sunblock every day to uncovered skin!

Beauty Secret

One of my best antiaging secrets couldn't be simpler: Wear sunglasses! Sunglasses can filter out UVA and UVB rays and protect your delicate eyelid skin from sun damage. Sunglasses could even lower your risk of UV-related eye cancer, such as melanoma of the eye (ouch!). They also prevent the need to squint, which may slow the formation of wrinkles. The bigger the sunglasses, the better. You probably wonder why Jacqueline Kennedy Onassis looked so young, even as she entered her sixties. I say it's because of those massive sunglasses! It probably wasn't her only beauty secret, but I'm sure it made a real difference.

For all these reasons, always wear sunglasses whenever you are in the sun. It helps if you have a pair stowed in your car for whenever you drive on a sunny day. Also start your children using sunglasses early to help get them in the habit as well. You're never too early to block the rays of the sun and prevent future wrinkles!

ABOUT SPF

Every bottle of sunscreen and sunblock tells you its SPF number. SPF stands for sun protection factor, and it applies to protection against only UVB rays, not UVA rays. For that reason, high-SPF sunscreen may prevent tanning and burning, but it may not protect you against premature aging, age spots, and wrinkles.

Insider Secret

Did you know there is a difference between sunscreen and sunblock? Sunscreen contains active chemicals that absorb the sun's ultraviolet rays. Mexoryl SX and stabilized avobenzone (Helioplex is good) are chemical sunscreens that provide good UVA protection, too. Chemical sunscreens must be applied more often because they wear off quickly.

Some postulate that chemical sunscreen is an endocrine disruptor, capable of disrupting hormonal balance. This can be especially concerning when applying it on children. Because of this, I recommend using physical sunblocks for children, not chemical sunscreens. Also, avoid using the popular aerosol sunscreen sprays on kids, as they are especially at risk of inhaling the chemicals. It may be easier to apply, but our children don't need to be breathing these chemicals into their developing lungs.

Sunblock physically blocks the sun's rays from reaching your skin. Sunblock ingredients are either titanium dioxide or zinc oxide. These minerals create a barrier. The problem with sunblock is that it can leave a white residue. If you don't like this, try a micronized physical sunblock, which is more expensive but looks nicer. However, most physical sunblocks are micronized now, and leave very little of a white residue behind.

Look for sunblocks or sunscreens labeled "broad spectrum," because then you know they also block out UVA. The FDA recently implemented a rule that a warning now be placed on sunscreens that lack adequate UVA protection. I also recommend an SPF of at least 30, which absorbs 97 percent of the sun's rays. The American Academy of Dermatology recommends a minimum SPF of 30, so they agree with me.

Q: *How much do you apply?*

SPF is based on the assumption that you are applying a good amount of sunblock on your skin. Most people don't apply nearly enough sunblock to be as effective as the SPF indicates. It's estimated that we apply only 25 percent of the recommended amount. Ideally, one ounce (or two tablespoons) of sunblock should be enough to cover the exposed parts of your body. This is the amount recommended by the American Academy of Dermatology. If you are bigger or have more area exposed (nudists, listen up!), then be more liberal—you'll need more than an ounce. Your face alone, including your ears and neck, should get at least a teaspoon. If you have short hair, apply sunscreen to your scalp, too, or look for a sunscreen spray made for hair.

Q: *When and how often to apply?*

If using a chemical sunscreen, apply it fifteen to thirty minutes prior to heading outdoors, to allow it to be absorbed by your skin. Reapply every two hours until you go indoors, more often if you are sweating or in the water. No sunscreen is truly waterproof! You need to reapply it after being in the water. Don't forget.

Also don't forget to apply sunscreen to your lips. Lips don't tan, so they are completely exposed to the effects of the sun. Use a lip balm with SPF 30 or higher, then apply your lip gloss or lipstick.

Q: *Which one to use?*

The best sunscreen or sunblock for you depends on your skin type. Follow this guide:

* **For sensitive skin:** Apply a physical sunblock and/or one that is fragrance free and hypoallergenic. Zinc oxide can soothe irritation and reduce redness in people who have sensitive skin or rosacea. The white color is worth it for you!

* **For acne-prone skin:** Use a gel-based, oil-free, or spray-on formula. Avoid heavy physical blockers. Avobenzone and oxybenzone (Neutrogena makes a combination

of avobenzone and oxybenzone that provides broad-spectrum UVA/UVB protection called Helioplex) are preferred for you.

* **For oily skin:** Avoid products with mineral oil. You may respond well to oil-free and spray-on products, just like people with acne-prone skin.

* **For dry skin:** Use lotion or cream formulas. These can contain aloe or other moisturizers. Avoid spray-on products that may contain drying alcohol.

Insider Tip

There is a sunscreen pill called **Heliocare** that you can buy over the counter. It is FDA-approved to aid in sun protection. If you are particularly fair-skinned, this may be an extra precaution that could benefit you. However, the sunscreen pill is not a substitute for sunblock or clothing. The pill begins to work thirty minutes after you take the dose.

Moisturizer

Sun protection is essential if you want to prevent premature aging, but the other big area that is important for protection of the skin is moisturizer. There are several kinds of moisturizers that can be used for various purposes, but in general, moisture makes skin more pliable, plump, young-looking, and resilient to damage like wrinkling. Moisturizer should be an important part of your skin-care routine, no matter what your skin type. Good moisturizers are most important in the winter, when the humidity drops in cooler climates and skin gets drier.

Most people need two different moisturizers: one that you apply in the morning that contains sunblock and possibly antioxidants to protect your skin during the day; and one that you apply at night that can renew and refresh your skin, such as Renova, or one with alpha-hydroxy acids to treat your skin. Let's look at some of the types:

Beauty Secret

If you have very cold winters, like we see in Michigan, make sure to use a humidifier, especially while you sleep. This can really help your skin stay hydrated. If your furnace has a humidifier attached to it, make sure it is set to "winter"; otherwise, it won't work.

OCCLUSIVES

Occlusive moisturizers prevent the loss of water from the skin. They provide a barrier so water doesn't seep out and evaporate. This keeps in the moisture you already have. Examples of occlusives are petroleum jelly, mineral oil, dimethicone, lanolin, shea butter, and beeswax. The problem with occlusives is that they can clog pores, leading to breakouts.

HUMECTANTS

Humectant moisturizers attract water from the air and from deep in the skin to the visible layer of skin. These moisturizers aren't as thick and heavy on the skin as occlusives, and they are less likely to clog pores, so they are better for people with acne issues. They plump the skin and reduce wrinkles, acting as instant wrinkle fillers. Some examples of humectants include hyaluronic acid, glycerin, lactic acid, propylene glycol, and urea.

In addition to these two types, moisturizers come in three forms:

1. Lotions are mostly water and the lightest (good for all skin types).

2. Creams are heavier and oilier than lotions (good for dry skin).

3. Ointments are the heaviest and oiliest (good for people with extremely dry skin).

Moisturizers may also contain many of the treatment elements we've already talked about in this chapter, such as antioxidants like vitamins C and E or green tea, retinoids, peptides, or growth factors, as well as SPF for protection. Use antioxidant moisturizers and moisturizers with an SPF during the day. It's best to apply moisturizers to the skin right after a shower and when your skin is still damp, in order to lock the moisture into your skin.

Beauty Secret

Frequently refresh your skin during the day with spritzes or sprays of spring water. This can help keep your skin moisturized, reducing the wrinkles that appear when the skin dries. Many skin-care companies, like La Roche-Posay, have small spray bottles that you can put in a bag or purse and use to keep your facial skin hydrated. I also like this company's moisturizer, **La Roche-Posay Anthelios**, which combines a humectant moisturizer with SPF.

At night, a more powerful moisturizer can help restore moisture to your skin and rejuvenate it. In addition to the moisturizing component, there are other ingredients to look for in a complete moisturizing night cream. Look for a retinoid to reverse aging while you sleep, such as retinol or Retin-A. Peptides and antioxidants can also fight off the aging process. Currently, my favorite night cream is **ZO Skin Health's Ommerse Overnight Recovery Cream**. Not only does it moisturize with a combination of occlusives and humectants, but it's also chock-full of other goodies like retinol and antioxidants.

YOUR AGE-FIX ROUTINE WRAP-UP

Find the products that work for you, and then stick with them—practicing your Age-Fix regimen on most days will make a real difference over time. Cleanse, treat, and protect every morning and every night, and in a month you'll be looking younger. If you want more guidance, I've put together individual Age-Fix routines for each skin type:

Applies to All Skin Types:

* During the day, protect your lips with a good lip balm that provides sun protection.

* In the evening, exfoliate your skin two to three times per week, right after cleansing.

* Morning and evening, apply a good eye cream.

For Dry Skin

Morning Routine:

1. Cleanse your skin with a hydrating cleanser, like **CeraVe Hydrating Cleanser**.
2. Treat your skin with a moisturizing antioxidant serum such as **ZO Medical Products C-Bright 10% Vitamin C**.
3. Protect your skin with a moisturizing sunblock (remember, the SPF must be at least 30!).

Evening Routine:

1. Cleanse your skin using the same hydrating cleanser.
2. Treat your skin with a retinol cream, which will be less drying than prescription-strength tretinoin. Try **Revision Retinol Facial Repair**. If your skin tolerates it, consider upgrading to a moisturizing version of tretinoin like **Renova** or **ReFissa**.
3. Protect your skin. If you are using Renova or ReFissa, you may not need a separate night cream. Those products may be moisturizing enough. If, however, you still have significant dryness, then use a peptide-based night cream such as **Olay Regenerist Night Recovery Cream**, which can be very hydrating and relatively cost-effective.

For Sensitive Skin

Morning Routine:

1. Cleanse your skin with a very mild hydrating cleanser, such as one that doesn't require rinsing, like **Avène Extremely Gentle Cleansing Lotion**. Follow this with a spritz of thermal spring water, such as **Avène Thermal Spring Water spray**.

2. Treat your skin with an antioxidant serum, such as **SkinCeuticals CE Ferulic**. If your skin is dry, then try a moisturizing version, such as the **ZO Medical Products C-Bright**.

3. Protect your skin with a fragrance-free physical sunblock that contains titanium dioxide or zinc oxide.

Evening Routine:

1. Cleanse your skin as you did in the morning.

2. Treat your skin with a growth factor–based cream, such as **SkinMedica TNS Essential Serum**, if your skin is too sensitive for retinoids.

3. Protect your skin with a fragrance-free night cream or moisturizer for sensitive skin. You can try various ones at your local department store to see what you like and tolerate–sensitive skin can be highly individual, and what bothers you may not bother someone else. I like the **Toleriane** line of moisturizers from **La Roche-Posay**. You might want to start by trying one of these.

For Normal/Combination Skin

Morning Routine:

1. Cleanse your skin with a gentle foaming cleanser like **Epionce Gentle Foaming Cleanser**, which will help to remove excess oil from your skin in addition to cleansing. If you have combination skin, then try a mild toner like **NARS Multi-Action Hydrating Toner** after cleansing. Use caution with alcohol-based toners, as they may be too drying for you.

2. Treat your skin with an antioxidant serum such as **SkinCeuticals CE Ferulic**.

3. Protect your skin with a gentle moisturizing sunblock.

Evening Routine:

1. Cleanse as you did in the morning.

2. Treat your skin with prescription-strength tretinoin (Retin-A). If you find it is too irritating, try a moisturizing version, such as **Renova** or **ReFissa**, which will be more moisturizing and may be less irritating.

3. Your tretinoin cream may suffice as your night cream, especially if you use Renova or ReFissa. However, if you are still experiencing some dryness, add a facial moisturizer. One of my favorites for normal or combination skin is **Teoxane RHA Serum**, which uses resilient hyaluronic acid to powerfully hydrate your skin but isn't thick or creamy like most night creams.

For Oily Skin

Morning Routine:

1. Cleanse your skin with a foaming cleanser that removes excess oil, such as **Neutrogena Fresh Foaming Cleanser**. Follow this up with an oil-reducing toner such as **ZO Medical Products Cebatrol Oil Control Pads**.

2. Treat your skin with an antioxidant serum that won't overmoisturize, such as **SkinCeuticals CE Ferulic**.

3. Protect your skin with an oil-free sunblock that won't clog your pores.

Evening Routine:

1. Cleanse your skin as you did in the morning.

2. Treat your skin with prescription-strength tretinoin. **Retin-A Micro** might be a good option to decrease irritation. Avoid versions of tretinoin like Renova and ReFissa. You don't need the extra moisturizing.

3. You could consider protecting your skin with a noncomedogenic (non-pore-clogging), gentle moisturizer. However, many people with oily skin don't need this step.

5 | THE AGE-FIX DIET

Wouldn't it be nice if looking younger were as easy as what you choose to put on your plate? Actually, to a large extent, this is true. What you eat actually alters the look and health of your skin, not just on your face but all over your body. The foods you choose can contribute to water weight gain, swelling, redness, acne, and the development of wrinkles, and can also affect skin tightness and elasticity, tissue firmness, and even how likely you are to get a sunburn.

Eating for a more youthful appearance isn't the same as eating for weight loss. Many diets will leave you looking thinner but older—more shrunken, wrinkled, droopy, or sallow. The dietary guidelines in this chapter, however, will do just the opposite. While you might very well lose a few extra pounds eating this way, you will definitely plump up your skin with hydration and moisture, strengthen and firm yourself all over with protein and collagen-building nutrients, and infuse your skin and body with antioxidants that fight the effects of aging and create a youthful bloom in your complexion. I'll urge you off the things that make you look older sooner: sugar, saturated fat, and simple carbohydrates. I'll also share with you tips on other lifestyle factors that may be making you look older, as well as those that could be helping you look younger.

For some of you, the suggestions in this chapter may represent a sea change in the way you look at food, eating, and maintaining your youth and health. It doesn't help that dietary recommendations over the past few decades have been very confusing. Are fats good or bad for you? What about carbohydrates? How about drinking wine?

I sympathize. I grew up in small-town America, where I was surrounded by fast-food restaurants and lots of processed food. As a kid, I remember riding my bike to the store and buying four candy bars for $1, then proceeding to plow through them over the following two days. In high school my friends and I would binge on oatmeal cream pies, French fries, and hamburgers. This contrasted severely with my parents' traditional Korean diet, which consisted of fish, vegetables, garlic, and white rice. Once I hit college, pizza and beer became new staples in my dietary routine. After marrying my wife and going through medical school, I began to reassess my diet. I reduced my visits to fast-food restaurants, limited the amount of red meat I ate, and almost completely cut out soft drinks in exchange for ice water.

Today, I'm aware that what I eat affects my health, my skin, and my youth more than ever. I've learned a lot from nutritionists, dietitians, and dermatologists, and yes, even some other surgeons (many surgeons have little nutritional training, but others make it an area of interest) about what foods can help us live longer, look better, and lead healthier lives. So please read on, as the suggestions in this chapter can make you look younger in as little as two weeks.

EATING FOR YOUTH

Those youthful-looking teenagers may survive on a diet of sugar and fast food, but if they keep it up, they won't be looking youthful for long. Young bodies can withstand a host of insults and still manage to look good for a few years, even a decade or so, but once you approach thirty, all that changes. You can't get away with the same dietary transgressions you used to take for granted, and the younger you are when you start eating for youth, the longer you will retain your youthful qualities.

As a general rule, the foods you already know are good for you, like vegetables, fruits, fish, whole grains, low-fat dairy, and lean protein, are the foods that also tend to promote antiaging and keep you looking younger longer. The foods you already know are bad for you, like sugar, saturated and trans fats, and processed junk foods, are the foods that actually cause accelerated skin aging. (I'll explain how this works later in this chapter.) However, you probably want more specifics, and indeed, there are very specific bad guys that are particularly likely to age you quickly, and some very specific good guys with super antiaging powers. Let's explore.

The Bad Guys: Foods That Age You

It's hard to give up your decadent favorites, but understanding what they do to you and your appearance may help, so let's start with the Most Wanted list of Youth-and-Beauty Bad Guys.

BAD GUY #1: SUGAR

Who can resist a warm chocolate chip cookie, a handful of candy from the candy jar, or a slice of cake with just the right thickness of frosting? You can, and should, because sugar is just about the worst thing you can eat when it comes to your skin. If there is one thing I would like you to take from this chapter, it's this:

Sugar = Wrinkles.

Let's look at why.

Just about everything you eat gets broken down into sugar. The process is complex, but to simplify, cookies, mashed potatoes, carrots, a sandwich, even a steak dinner, gets converted into glucose (a type of simple sugar) for your body to use as energy. Anything you don't need right away gets stored in your liver and muscles in the form of glycogen, which your body can use later when it needs more energy. Foods with more carbohydrates are more readily turned into sugar to fuel the body than foods with more protein and/or fat (this is why athletes sometimes "carb-load" before a race or competition). If you take in excessive calories and your liver and muscles have all the glycogen you need, anything left over gets stored in your fat cells. The more sugar you eat, the more likely you will have significant stores of body fat, because your body has to put that excess sugar somewhere.

However, the problem when it comes to health, as well as beauty, isn't so much about fat as it is about insulin. Normally, when you eat food and your body turns it into glucose, your blood sugar goes up. In response, your body releases just enough insulin to help shuttle that extra sugar into the liver, muscles, and fat cells. When you eat too much sugar, however (and that can mean too many calories, especially carbohydrate calories made of starchy and sugary foods), your body can't keep up. A large amount of sugar (including the sugar from refined carbohydrates like white bread) triggers the body to release a flood of insulin to get that blood sugar down before it hurts you. This in turn can push blood sugar too low. Too much of this up-and-down blood sugar and insulin instability can lead to diabetes and many other related issues, including obesity and system-wide inflammation. Chronic inflammation damages your skin and impedes your body's natural processes, which can lead to compromised health over time. As you probably already know, glowing health looks younger. Ill health looks (and feels!) older. As a final insult, spiking insulin levels can also result in increased levels of androgenic hormones and excess oil, worsening acne.

Sugar spikes

↓

Insulin spikes

Diabetes   Obesity   Inflammation   Worsening acne

SUGAR SPIKES

But perhaps the most direct link between sugar and aging is glycation. High levels of sugar in the bloodstream cause a chain reaction of accelerated aging when sugar molecules bond to protein and fat molecules in the body, deforming and stiffening them. This happens with glucose, and at an even higher rate with fructose (high-fructose corn syrup, a sweetener that's very common in processed foods, is one of the worst "foods" in terms of premature skin aging—avoid it like poison!). The molecules that are impacted by glycation include collagen and elastin, which are the building blocks of your skin. Collagen and elastin give skin its firmness and elasticity, but when sugar molecules attach to them, they get stiff, bent out of shape, and drained of color. They become sugar-protein hybrids, called advanced glycation end products or (appropriately) AGEs. And they aren't pretty.

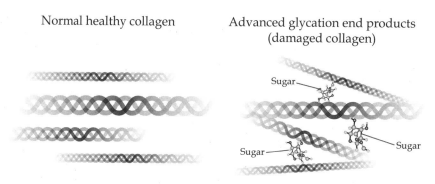

GLYCATION

Glycation is a natural process and some AGEs are inevitable, but the more AGEs you have, the more your skin will be affected, even overwhelmed. The equation is simple: Too much sugar = too many AGEs. This can result in premature wrinkles, sagging, stiffness, slower cell turnover, and a loss of circulation to the skin. It can cause unattractive distribution of fat pockets and a loss of that youthful bloom. All skin ages eventually, but AGEs have a definite accelerating effect that becomes most noticeable after the age of thirty-five.

This is all some people need to know to cut out the sweet stuff, but sugar and simple carbohydrates are hard to resist. Overeating, which creates a flood of glucose, and especially overeating high-sugar and high-starch foods (from candy to white rice), is the quickest way to age due to too many AGEs, so the next time you are tempted to eat too many carbohydrates, just picture your skin and the damage you could cause by eating that extra slice of cake.

Another aging effect of sugar is inflammation. Many studies have linked high blood sugar and also the high insulin that inevitably follows to system-wide chronic inflammation, which can cause chronic disease but can also have a negative effect on a youthful appearance. Chronic inflammation can worsen rosacea and rashes, can increase skin oiliness, and may also weaken the collagen and elastin in your skin over time.

While inflammation can be useful in skin-care treatments (for example, chemical peels create an "injury," and the healing of the skin improves the skin's appearance via rejuvenation), chronic inflammation can impair the skin's natural healing ability, slowly degrading skin quality and accelerating aging. Antioxidants can be an effective treatment for inflammation. I'll talk about these later in this chapter.

Even if you weren't at all worried about wrinkles, sugar has also been linked to acne. When high blood sugar spikes trigger insulin spikes, insulin triggers insulin-like growth factor-1 (IGF-1). Both insulin and IGF-1 increase the production of androgens, which are hormones that can trigger acne.[17] The short version: Sugar accelerates aging and causes breakouts—two strong reasons to pass on the sweet stuff.

Caution!

Guess what one food or beverage item will age you the most? Soda pop! A recent study suggests that intake of these sugar-sweetened drinks actually impacts cellular aging by shrinking the length of the caps on the ends of your chromosomes, called telomeres, which are associated with cellular regeneration and, by association, longevity.[18] Just one twenty-ounce sugary soda every day could mean 4.6 fewer years to live—a life-shortening effect equal to that of smoking! This is just one more very good reason never to drink soda pop.

If you follow the diet industry at all, you have probably heard of the glycemic index, or GI. This is a measure of how quickly a particular food gets converted into glucose in your bloodstream after you eat it, and it can help you to choose the best carbohydrates. The GI scale goes from 0 to 100. Pure glucose has a GI of 100. A bagel has a GI of 72, an apple has a GI of 39, chickpeas have a GI of 10, and peanuts have a GI of 7. The GI of foods can also be influenced by ripeness and cooking method, as well as what you eat them with. A high-GI food eaten with fat, for example, will not be absorbed as quickly.

Foods with a high GI (baked potatoes, white rice, white bread, processed breakfast cereal, many processed packaged foods) create glucose quickly and are more likely to cause a blood sugar spike and then an insulin spike; they can also cause cellular inflammation, especially if you eat a lot of them. Refined grains are the worst offenders. The process of refining grains, such as wheat flour, involves removing the bran and germ.

That takes away the fiber, as well as many essential nutrients, and fiber slows down the release of sugar from the grain. The result is a lighter, less bulky product (think white bread versus whole-grain bread), which is why white flour products like white bread, bagels, and croissants as well as other refined grains like white rice are high on the GI scale.

Foods with a low GI (beans, seeds, nuts, whole grains, and some fruits) take more time to digest and release glucose into your bloodstream more gradually. These keep blood sugar and insulin more even, because these foods contain a lot of fiber, protein, and/or fat. Several recent diets have encouraged a focus on low-GI foods as a method of weight loss, because blood sugar spikes and dips can encourage overeating. Because of the effect of sugar on the skin, I believe that paying attention to the GI of the foods you eat is also an excellent method for maintaining a youthful appearance.

Glycemic load (GL) is another useful term. While the GI measures how quickly a food is broken down into glucose in the liver, the GL takes into account how many carbohydrates are in an individual serving size. Some foods can have a high GI, but because there aren't very many of those high-GI carbs in a serving of a particular food, it can have a low GL, and therefore not have that much of an impact on your blood sugar. For example, pancakes and sweet potatoes have a similar glycemic index, but a serving of sweet potatoes has a much lower glycemic load than a serving of white-flour pancakes with syrup.

For these reasons, one of the best ways to eat for youth is to choose moderate portions of low-GI foods and/or low-GL foods. These are digested more slowly and release sugar into the bloodstream more gradually. This gives the body a chance to keep up with the glucose coming in. There aren't large sugar spikes, which means there aren't large insulin spikes. The blood sugar / insulin waves stay nice and even, and that's what you want. You want your body to use the glucose you take in, rather than flood it with more than it can handle.

Unfortunately, most foods don't currently include GI or GL values on the package. You have to know them or look them up online. There are many GI and GL food lists out there, so you can always look them up, but most people aren't going to do that regularly. Instead, take a good look once at a few lists to get a general idea of the kinds of foods that have high and low GI and GL values, and then you will get the basic idea. One good source is the Harvard Medical School's list "Glycemic Index and Glycemic Load for 100+ Foods." Check out their website.[19] Also remember that fiber, protein, and fat always slow down the release of glucose, so never eat simple carbs alone. Add some almond butter to your bagel, some milk to your cereal, some chicken to your pasta, and a small handful of peanuts to go with that candy you grab from the office candy jar.

Caution!

Diet isn't the only thing that can trigger accelerated aging. Consider these other controllable lifestyle factors:

* **Smoking:** A study on twins by Case Western Reserve University found that smoking removes 2.5 years from your life for every decade you smoke.[20] This number may be even higher if you smoke heavily and/or add other vices like heavy drinking, other drugs, and a lot of time in the sun.

* **Stress:** Temporary stress can be a good thing. When your brain believes your body is under threat, it signals the release of hormones like adrenaline, cortisol, and other corticosteroids to make you faster and stronger, increase your reaction time, elevate your sensory perceptions, and help you respond effectively to emergencies. Chronic stress, however, has a more insidious effect. Those stress hormones aren't meant to be circulating in your bloodstream all the time, and when they do, they can cause widespread inflammation that leads to premature aging, as well as putting you at greater risk for dangerous health issues like heart disease.

* **Sleep deprivation:** Your body undergoes major repairs while you sleep, including repairs to your skin. If you skimp on sleep, not only will you be more susceptible to stress and more likely to crave sugar, but your skin will be less likely to repair itself from the damage of the previous day (from sun, dry air, and chemical assaults from without and within). Try to get at least seven hours of sleep every night–and remember to sleep on your back when you can, to minimize the time your face spends sagging from gravity and creased by your pillow.

* **Menopause:** Okay, you can't exactly control menopause, but the drop in estrogen that happens during this time in life reduces collagen, causing skin to thin and wrinkle. Hormonal changes can also increase dryness and shrink fat pockets under the skin, and this can all lead to sagging and wrinkles. These hormone changes can also cause an increase in spider veins, broken capillaries (called telangiectasias), and wrinkles. Fortunately, a good skin-care regimen and a diet rich in antioxidants and soy protein can help to combat some of these effects.

BAD GUY #2: SATURATED AND TRANS FATS

The next youth wreckers are saturated and trans fats. There is a lot in the media right now about fat and how it isn't as bad as we thought, but there are different kinds of fats, and they have different kinds of effects on health and, especially, on aging. Saturated and trans fats in particular are more damaging to the skin than healthier fats like monounsaturated and polyunsaturated fats.

A study in the *Journal of the American College of Nutrition* found that people who ate a lot of butter, margarine, and foods high in saturated fats (like fatty processed meat, cakes, and pastries) had more wrinkling than those who ate less.[21] We also know that animal proteins that are also high in saturated fat increase inflammation in the body.

These include fatty cuts of beef and pork, dark meat poultry, and high-fat cured meats like sausage, bacon, and bologna (cured meat also contains additional inflammation-causing substances).

Trans fat consumption puts you in another danger zone. Trans fats, or trans fatty acids, are industrially modified plant oils that are cheap and don't tend to spoil quickly, so they are widely used in processed foods and fried fast food. You can spot them by the term *partially hydrogenated vegetable oil* on food packaging. Although they were once used widely, the FDA has now determined that these fats are not safe. We know they raise the bad (LDL) cholesterol and depress the good (HDL) cholesterol, increasing the risk of heart disease, stroke, and diabetes. They are also pro-inflammatory and accelerate the aging process. I do not recommend you consume any amount at all. There is no safe minimum.

BAD GUY #3: SALT

Your body needs some salt, but most people eat way too much, which can cause your body to retain water. This results in puffy eyelids, bags under your eyes, and festoons (those saggy droopy folds and puffy areas that accumulate beneath your eyes, even down to your cheeks). Too much salt can also result in swollen legs, ankles, arms, and wrists. It's not pretty and it's not good for your blood pressure. The biggest source of salt in most people's diets is from packaged, processed food (like canned soup) and restaurant food (especially fast food, but most restaurants go heavy on the salt). Eat at home more often and use just enough salt in your cooking to satisfy you. Salting your food isn't nearly as bad as eating, for example, a bag of fast-food French fries or a can of chicken noodle soup.

The Good Guys: Foods That Fight Aging

Now that you understand the dietary culprits for premature aging and some of the foods to avoid, let's look at all the dietary good guys. Because aren't we all more interested in what we get to eat, rather than what we shouldn't eat? Fortunately, there are many delicious and satisfying foods that not only can fill you up and make you feel good but also are full of antiaging compounds to keep you looking younger longer. These are your dietary superstars, and the meal plan at the end of the chapter includes the foods on this list.

GOOD GUY #1: ANTIOXIDANTS

You already know that topical antioxidants like vitamin C fight free radicals on the surface of your skin, but foods rich in antioxidants can do the same thing from the inside. Antioxidant-rich foods can even help protect you from the harmful UV rays of the sun and the free radicals they can generate. In fact, some doctors believe that eating antioxidants is even more effective in reducing free-radical damage created by UV rays than applying topical antioxidants.

Antioxidants are substances that prevent cell damage from free radicals. I explained how this worked in the previous chapter, but just as a reminder, free radicals are unstable molecules that are missing an electron. They seek to steal electrons from healthy cells, causing damage. They can be generated by natural metabolism in the body but can also come into the body via pollution, chemicals, and exposure to sunlight. They can also be generated in greater numbers when the body is under stress. Antioxidants are substances like vitamins C and E that carry an extra electron. They donate this to the free radical, neutralizing its scavenging and damaging action. Let's look at some of the best ones for good eating.

Vitamin C: One of the great things about vitamin C, in addition to its free radical–fighting power, is its essential role in the production of collagen and elastin. That's why vitamin C is so good for your skin, whether you eat it or apply it topically. Vitamin C is water soluble, so it is quickly excreted by your body. In other words, you don't store it, so you should eat vitamin C–rich foods every day. A study from the UK found that women with a higher vitamin C intake had fewer wrinkles and less dry skin than women with average or low levels of vitamin C intake.[22] While most people think of citrus fruits as the best source of vitamin C, many fruits and vegetables contain lots of it, especially when you eat them fresh. Vitamin C degrades quickly after harvest and with cooking, so eat these fruits and veggies as soon as you can after purchasing, and look for them in the farmers' market, where they are more likely to be extremely fresh.

Try to eat at least two servings of vitamin C–rich food every day. That's about a cup of berries or chopped raw vegetables.

Good sources include:

* Blackberries
* Blueberries
* Broccoli
* Brussels sprouts
* Cabbage
* Cantaloupe
* Cauliflower
* Gooseberries
* Grapefruit
* Honeydew
* Kale
* Kiwifruit

- * Mangoes
- * Oranges
- * Papaya
- * Pineapple
- * Pomegranates
- * Raspberries

- * Red bell peppers
- * Rhubarb
- * Strawberries
- * Sweet potatoes
- * Tomatoes

Caution!

A study in the journal *Free Radical Biology and Medicine* showed that the protein in milk blocks the action of antioxidants in blueberries.[23] Enjoy blueberries with nondairy milk or yogurt (like those made from soy or almond milk), or eat them alone for the best antiaging effect.

Vitamin E: This antioxidant vitamin is excellent at protecting the skin from UV radiation as well as preventing free-radical damage. Unlike water-soluble vitamin C, vitamin E is fat soluble. That means your body can store it in fat tissue, so it isn't as important to get some every day, and it is unusual for someone living in the United States to have a vitamin E deficiency. However, vitamin E has many benefits, so enjoy vitamin E–rich foods when you have the opportunity.

Some good choices include:

- * Almonds
- * Anchovies
- * Avocados
- * Broccoli
- * Butternut squash
- * Carrots
- * Dried apricots
- * Hazelnuts
- * Olive oil

- * Peanuts
- * Pine nuts
- * Pumpkin
- * Salmon (smoked salmon has even more)
- * Shrimp
- * Silken tofu
- * Spinach
- * Sunflower seeds
- * Wheat germ

Vitamin A: Vitamin A is another fat-soluble vitamin with antioxidant action, and many skin-care products contain a form of vitamin A (retinoids like retinol and tretinoin). Technically, vitamin A is actually a group of compounds, including both retinoids and carotenoids. Retinoids have anti-inflammatory effects but are often found in foods high in saturated fat and cholesterol, like egg yolks, shrimp, and liver.

Beta-carotene is a carotenoid that the body can convert to a usable form of vitamin A. Fruits and vegetables that are a deep yellow or orange color are typically rich in beta-carotene, and the effect in the body is most pronounced when those orange vegetables, like carrots and sweet potatoes, are cooked. Beta-carotene increases the production of collagen and glycosaminoglycans, which improve the skin's ability to retain moisture. This can prevent dry, scaling, cracked skin. There is some evidence that beta-carotene supplements may have some hazardous effects, although this seems to be most pronounced in smokers. Just in case, get your beta-carotene from foods—it's easy to do.

Try to get both retinoids and beta-carotene in your diet. Retinoids are more readily absorbed, and beta-carotene has to be converted, but beta-carotene also confers other antioxidant benefits, such as being particularly good for your eyes (which is why your mother told you to eat your carrots).

Good sources of retinoids include:

* Cheese

* Eggs

* Fish (especially tuna, trout, herring, cod, salmon, and mackerel)

* Liver

* Milk (lower-fat varieties contain more retinol)

* Shrimp

Good sources of beta-carotene include:

* Apricots (especially dried)

* Cantaloupe

* Carrots

* Dark green, leafy vegetables (like kale and spinach—not orange, but they contain a lot of beta-carotene)

* Mangoes

* Nectarines

* Papaya

* Peaches

* Pumpkin (canned pumpkin is a great source)

* Sweet potatoes

* Winter squashes like butternut and acorn

Carotenoids: There are many different kinds of carotenoids, many of which do not convert to vitamin A like beta-carotene does, but that have profound antioxidant and anti-inflammatory effects. They include substances like lycopene, lutein, and zeaxanthin. Lycopene, found in red vegetables and fruits like watermelon, tomatoes, and red peppers, is perhaps one of the most potent of the free radical–destroying antioxidants, and cooked tomatoes are the best source. Canned tomato sauce and tomato paste are easy ways to get a good dose of lycopene, which is even better absorbed if you combine it with a little fat, because it is fat soluble—which also makes it more delicious. Add olive oil to your pasta sauce and extra sauce with your pizza—it's good for your skin!

In fact, lycopene is especially effective in reversing damage to the skin. There is even some evidence that eating a lot of tomatoes and tomato products can prevent sunburn. A recent presentation of research at the Royal Society of Medicine in London[24] revealed that participants who added 5 tablespoons of tomato paste per day to their normal diet showed a 33 percent reduced risk of sunburn after twelve weeks! Another recent study demonstrated that women who took lycopene, soy, and vitamin C supplements for six months showed significant improvement in fine lines, skin elasticity, and skin radiance.[25]

The carotenoids lutein and zeaxanthin have also been shown to help protect the skin from UV exposure. They are both antioxidants that can be found in the eye, where they filter out damaging blue waves and act to neutralize free radicals. They are essential to eye health, but the skin also contains lutein and zeaxanthin, where they also prevent damage and help to maintain the structural integrity of the skin. These carotenoids are most prevalent in cooked green, leafy vegetables but can also be found in some other foods.

The best sources of lutein and zeaxanthin include:

* Collard greens

* Corn

* Egg yolks

* Grapes

* Kale

* Kiwifruit

* Orange juice
* Orange peppers
* Spinach

* Turnip greens
* Zucchini and other squashes[26]

The bottom line is that antioxidants are easy to get in your diet as long as you eat a variety of colorful fruits and vegetables. Just taking an antioxidant supplement like vitamin C isn't enough to fight the free-radical onslaught of modern life. Foods are much better sources of absorbable and usable antioxidants, as they contain many different beneficial antioxidants like polyphenols and flavonoids that also help to neutralize free radicals. (These are UV-protective antioxidants that inhibit inflammation and tissue damage, found in onions, dark chocolate, soy, cherries, red wine, green tea, and whole grains.) You can't get that whole package in a supplement.

Beauty Secret

Green tea may just be the most powerful of all antioxidant sources. Green tea contains polyphenols that scavenge free radicals and protect against photo damage. A 1997 presentation of University of Kansas research at the American Chemical Society national meeting found that antioxidants in green tea called catechins (a phenol) are more than 100 times more effective at neutralizing free radicals than vitamin C, and 25 times more powerful than vitamin E.[27] Green tea is also chock-full of the amino acid L-theanine, which, when combined with caffeine, has been shown in studies to increase relaxation, concentration, and focus. Many people find that it helps to improve their ability to stay calm and focused throughout the morning. Not a bad way to start the day!

The ideal amount for better skin with fewer wrinkles and more luster is four cups per day, although you can still benefit from two to three cups if the caffeine makes you jittery. Add lemon juice for even more antioxidants. If you don't like green tea, you could also take 500 mg per day of a green tea supplement.

GOOD GUY #2: OMEGA-3 FATTY ACIDS

There is a lot of conflicting information out there about fats and which ones are good or bad for you and how much and what percentage you need of which ones. I won't put myself in the center of the debate about whether saturated fats or polyunsaturated industrial seed oils are the true culprits of inflammation, but I will say this: Whenever you can, avoid saturated fats, trans fats, and highly processed industrial fats like corn oil and soybean oil, and eat more of the good natural fats we know for sure help elevate good cholesterol, moisturize the skin, reduce inflammation, and help you look younger:

* Monounsaturated fats like those in olive oil, walnuts, and avocados.

* The polyunsaturated fat known as omega-3 fatty acid, which can be further subdivided into eicosapentaenoic acid (EPA) and docosahexaenoic acid (DHA), found in cold-water fish like salmon, tuna, and sardines; and alpha-linolenic acid (ALA), found in flaxseed, chia seeds, canola oil, and soy products like tofu. The body converts ALA to the more usable EPA and DHA.

Whereas other types of fats tend to be inflammatory, monounsaturated fats and omega-3 fats tend to be anti-inflammatory. They soothe and calm inflamed, broken-out skin. They decrease the redness and damage associated with UV exposure. Even though they are not antioxidants, they fight free-radical damage. They also improve skin elasticity, resulting in fewer wrinkles.

The easiest ways to incorporate more omega-3s is to eat fish as your protein whenever you can—aim for fish as a dinner entrée two or three times per week. You could also take 1000 mg of fish oil per day in supplement form. For more ALAs, add ground flaxseed, chia seeds, or walnuts to your oatmeal or yogurt. For more monounsaturated fats, use olive oil instead of butter for flavoring your food. A good-quality extra-virgin olive oil tastes delicious on whole-grain toast (which has a lower GI value than white toast).

Good sources of monounsaturated fatty acids include:

* Almond butter
* Almond oil
* Almonds
* Canola oil (a source of both monounsaturated and polyunsaturated fatty acids)
* Hazelnut oil
* Hazelnuts
* Macadamia nuts
* Olive oil
* Olives
* Peanut butter
* Safflower oil
* Sesame oil
* Sesame seeds

Good sources of omega-3 fatty acids, including EPA, DHA, and ALA, include:

* Chia seeds
* Cod
* Flaxseed (ground) or flaxseed oil
* Grass-fed beef
* Halibut
* Hemp seed oil

* Herring
* Mackerel
* Oysters
* Salmon (wild-caught only)
* Sardines

* Seaweed
* Tofu
* Trout
* Tuna (fresh)
* Walnuts

GOOD GUY #3: ZINC

Our last dietary superstar is zinc. Zinc is a mineral that helps to create more efficient collagen turnover and improves skin's rejuvenation rate. It also acts as an antioxidant and boosts cell growth and repair. Many fish with high omega-3 fatty acids also contain zinc. Other good sources of zinc include:

* Beef
* Cashews
* Cocoa powder
* Crab
* Garbanzo beans
* Lamb
* Lentils
* Lobster
* Oysters (cooked)

* Pork (lean)
* Pumpkin seeds
* Quinoa
* Sesame seeds
* Shrimp
* Spinach
* Turkey
* Wheat germ

WHAT TO EAT

You've got a lot of information, but how do you implement it? Here are some helpful strategies for increasing your intake of the Good Guys while decreasing your reliance on the Bad Guys:

* **Go whole grain.** Whenever you have a choice, choose whole grains over refined grains. Change your white toast to whole-wheat toast. Change white rice to brown rice. Choose whole-grain cereals or oatmeal instead of refined sugary cereals. Try

whole-grain pasta, including brown-rice pasta, instead of the white stuff. Be aware that many products will advertise themselves as "whole grain" or "multigrain" or "whole wheat" but will actually contain only a small amount of whole grain compared to refined grain. This is especially common with bread products, including bagels, English muffins, and hamburger buns. Read the label. The whole-grain ingredients should be listed first. Ideally, the product will contain 100 percent whole grains. Popcorn is a whole grain, so snack on that whenever you need something crunchy. Just don't drown it in butter and salt.

* **Use protein.** If you decide to eat a food with a high glycemic index, such as something with sugar or white flour, always pair it with protein to slow down the release of glucose in your bloodstream. For example, have a hard-boiled egg with your waffle, put lean steak in your stir-fry, or have almonds with your raisins.

* **Go green.** If you are a coffee drinker, try alternating a cup of coffee with a cup of green tea. You'll still get the caffeine boost you crave, but you'll also get powerful antioxidants. Coffee has antioxidants, too, but green tea has different ones that are particularly skin friendly. Peppermint tea is another good option, since it is also full of antioxidants that slow down aging of the skin.

* **Spice (and herb) it up.** Many herbs, spices, and seasonings also contain potent antioxidants, so use them liberally, especially the spices cinnamon (skip the sugar), cloves, cumin, curry powder, turmeric, and saffron, and the herbs basil, lemon balm, marjoram, oregano, peppermint, rosemary, sage, tarragon, and thyme. Use herbs and spices liberally when cooking, sprinkle fresh herbs on salads or sandwiches, and add a shake of cinnamon to your coffee or tea to fight off wrinkles and aging!

* **Pass on the processed food.** Anything that comes in a package is suspect, but baked goods and snack foods are the worst—cupcakes, cookies, donuts, and kids' cereals contain refined flour and too much sugar, which will spike your blood sugar and your insulin levels. Fried foods like chips and crackers are often loaded with salt and fat, and may contain trans fats. Beware of so-called healthy versions of your favorite snacks, too. Low-fat versions often contain an extra load of sugar (this can be especially true for peanut butter), and even whole-grain snacks may contain too much sugar, salt, and fat.

* **Start your day with fruit.** A plate of fruit every morning is a great way to load up on antioxidants without fat, salt, or added sugar. My father eats a plate of fruit every morning, and I suspect that man is going to live to be a hundred.

* **Satisfy your sweet tooth with dark chocolate.** Chocolate is graded according to how much raw cocoa it contains. The higher the percentage of raw cocoa, the greater the antioxidant activity. Look for chocolate with at least 70 percent cocoa for maximum antioxidants and minimum added sugar. I like the 85 percent cocoa chocolate. Several brands make an 85 percent chocolate bar, including Lindt, Green and Black, Ghirardelli (86 percent), and Endangered Species (88 percent). Hershey's bars, chocolate kisses, and dark-chocolate versions of your favorite candy like Special Dark, dark-chocolate M&M'S, and dark-chocolate Raisinets, as well as anything made of milk chocolate, don't have enough raw cocoa to be beneficial, so skip them. They are mostly sugar.

* **Remember: green, yellow, orange, red.** The most antioxidant-rich foods are brightly colored.

* **Eat more protein.** Protein provides the building blocks of collagen, and your body needs it to repair and replace collagen that has degraded with age or that is damaged by free radicals. One study showed that women with lower protein intake had more wrinkles than women with higher protein intake.[28] The USDA recommends 0.8–1.0 grams of protein per kilogram of body weight per day. For example, a 150-pound (68.2 kg) woman would require about 68 grams of protein per day.

* **Drink up!** Water is extremely important for hydration. Everything in your body will work better when you are well hydrated, and the more you drink, the more you will moisturize your skin from the inside. If you are chronically dehydrated (and many people are), drinking eight glasses of water a day can make you look younger almost immediately.

Beauty Secret

A glass of red wine each day might be one of the best and most enjoyable things you can do for your health and appearance. Health experts have been drinking red wine as far back as Hippocrates, the Greek physician who drank wine as part of what he believed to be a healthy diet (he also used wine as a disinfectant). Back in 1991, a piece on the show *60 Minutes* first popularized the notion of the "French Paradox," asking why the French, who traditionally ate a large amount of high-fat and heavy-dairy foods, had such a low rate of cardiovascular disease. One theory was the red wine. Could something in red wine, which the French drink moderately but enthusiastically, combat the ill effects of an otherwise decadent diet?

Twenty years later, we know that red wine does indeed include antioxidants, primarily polyphenols, the most potent of which is resveratrol. This comes from the skin of the grapes, which are highly concentrated in red wine (which is why both grape juice and white wine don't contain as much–these beverages are in contact with the grape skins for much less time than red wine). Laboratory studies have shown the antiaging effects of resveratrol on animals, but there still are no large-scale scientific studies of resveratrol's effects on humans. There is also little evidence that resveratrol supplements do as much good as drinking actual red wine.

However, there are studies showing that red wine does have positive effects, including improving the balance between bad (LDL) and good (HDL) cholesterols, easing platelet aggregation that can predispose people to strokes and heart disease, lowering the risk of developing Alzheimer's disease and dementia, decreasing the risk of diabetes and high blood sugar, and lowering the risk of precancerous skin lesions. Also, interestingly, the IQs of wine drinkers were reported to be eighteen points higher than those of beer drinkers.[29] However, like most things, red wine should be taken in moderation. One glass with dinner is plenty. Don't drink the whole bottle, no matter how good it tastes! Overindulging in wine is actually more damaging to health and skin than not drinking at all. It can make you look and feel older due to the dehydrating and other toxic effects of too much alcohol.

One caution: If you tend to have an alcohol flush reaction due to the histamines in red wine, causing your eczema or rosacea to flare up, then red wine isn't for you. Some Asians can't tolerate wine or any other type of alcoholic drink, due to a condition known as aldehyde dehydrogenase deficiency. Even a sip of alcohol causes their faces, and sometimes their entire bodies, to flush beet-red. Not a fun party trick! If alcohol makes you flush, it's best to get your antioxidants in other ways.

For maximum antioxidant benefit, pair a glass of wine with a square of dark chocolate. This is my wife Amy's favorite combination. Now, that's a prescription I bet you can get excited about!

YOUR TWO-WEEK AGE-FIX MEAL PLAN

If you like a little more guidance in your diet, try this meal plan, which combines many of the suggestions in this chapter into a nutrient-dense, youth-enhancing, antiaging diet plan. This plan isn't about weight loss, so I'm not giving you portion sizes. If you are trying to lose weight, keep your portions of starchy, sugary, and fatty foods smaller (½ cup of grains, 1 piece of sweet fruit, 3 or 4 ounces of meat), but load up on the vegetables and low-GI fruits (like berries), and you may be surprised at how quickly antiaging foods also turn into weight-loss foods.

Note that this meal plan includes two snacks. Snacks are helpful for keeping blood sugar and insulin on an even keel, which is one of our goals. If you get hungry between meals, have a snack. This can help you eat less during your main meals. Remember that eating large portions, even of low-GI foods, can spike blood sugar. If snacks help, go for it. If you find that snacks just keep you thinking about food more often and don't impact how much you eat at a meal, then skip them.

WEEK ONE

MONDAY

Breakfast:
Oatmeal with blueberries, walnuts, and nondairy milk (like almond or soy milk), green tea

Snack:
Mango slices and raw almonds

Lunch:
Lentil soup over brown rice

Snack:
Low-fat cottage cheese with pineapple cubes

Dinner:
Lean steak topped with sautéed bell peppers, mushrooms, and onions, romaine salad with olive-oil vinaigrette, baked sweet potato with olive oil

TUESDAY

Breakfast:
Two scrambled eggs with chopped onions, spinach or kale, and tomatoes, fruit smoothie made with blueberries or strawberries, orange juice, and crushed ice

Snack:
Carrots and hummus

Lunch:
Spinach salad with grilled chicken, oranges, and walnuts

Snack:
Greek yogurt with strawberries and cinnamon

Dinner:
Shrimp skewers over brown rice with olive oil, red wine (optional)

WEDNESDAY

Breakfast:
Whole-grain or sprouted-grain toast with almond butter, fresh orange or grapefruit, green tea

Snack:
Smoked salmon with capers on whole-grain crackers

Lunch:
Tuna salad on whole-grain toast, corn and black bean salad

Snack:
Popcorn without butter or added salt–or if you are really adventurous, try roasted seaweed like my mom makes! (Go easy on the salt.)

Dinner:
Taco salad with romaine lettuce, ground turkey, black beans, fresh tomato salsa, low-fat or nonfat sour cream, a sprinkle of low-fat cheese, and baked tortilla chips

THURSDAY

Breakfast:
Turkey sausage and poached egg on whole-grain English muffin with low-fat Swiss cheese, fruit smoothie made with half a banana, strawberries, crushed ice, and a little water or coconut water

Snack:
Olives and goat cheese

Lunch:
Homemade veggie chili made with tomato sauce, beans, lots of veggies, and garnished with avocado cubes

Snack:
Apple with peanut butter (I personally love peanut butter!)

Dinner:
Whole-grain spaghetti with marinara sauce, a few turkey meatballs, roasted asparagus with olive oil and lemon juice, red wine (optional)

FRIDAY

Breakfast:
Nonfat Greek yogurt with pumpkin puree or applesauce, chopped dried apricots, and hazelnuts, green tea

Snack:
Avocado on whole-grain toast

Lunch:
Romaine salad with salmon and sliced almonds, olive oil–based dressing

Snack:
Whole-grain tortilla with tomato sauce and low-fat mozzarella cheese, broiled

Dinner:
Butternut squash soup garnished with toasted pine nuts, whole-grain bread with olive oil

SATURDAY

Breakfast:
Whole-grain waffle topped with almond butter and sliced strawberries or peaches, green tea

Snack:
Peach or nectarine and sunflower seeds

Lunch:
Whole-grain bagel with hummus and lots of veggies, pear

Snack:
Whole-grain cereal with nondairy or nonfat milk

Dinner:
Roasted salmon, roasted Brussels sprouts, cubed winter squash with olive oil

SUNDAY

Breakfast:
Spinach mushroom omelet with crumbled goat cheese, mixed berries, green tea

Snack:
Greek yogurt with chia seeds and strawberries

Lunch:
Butternut squash soup topped with Greek yogurt, small spinach salad

Snack:
Cantaloupe with cottage cheese

Dinner:
Roast chicken (don't eat the skin), mashed potatoes made with low-fat milk and olive oil, green salad with olive-oil vinaigrette

WEEK TWO

MONDAY

Breakfast:
Oatmeal with chopped dried apricots, almonds, and cinnamon, skim or nondairy milk, and green tea

Snack:
Blackberries with Greek yogurt

Lunch:
Tuna salad sandwich with lettuce and tomato

Snack:
Whole-grain crackers with almond butter

Dinner:
Shrimp stir-fry with all your favorite veggies over brown rice

TUESDAY

Breakfast:
Omelet with goat cheese, sautéed red and green peppers, and onions, green tea

Snack:
Broccoli florets with hummus

Lunch:
Vegetable soup, hummus and whole-grain crackers

Snack:
Baked tortilla chips with fresh salsa

Dinner:
Roasted salmon, shredded cabbage and carrots with olive-oil vinaigrette, red wine (optional)

WEDNESDAY

Breakfast:
Smoothie made with nonfat Greek yogurt, pumpkin puree, pecans, flaxseed, and real maple syrup, green tea

Snack:
Leftover shredded cabbage and carrots with olive-oil vinaigrette

Lunch:
Tomato soup with grilled cheese on whole-grain bread

Snack:
Orange and pistachios

Dinner:
Tostadas or tacos with corn tortillas, mashed pinto beans, chopped tomatoes, lettuce, guacamole, and salsa

THURSDAY

Breakfast:
Sweet potatoes sautéed with kale and onions, poached egg, green tea

Snack:
Dried apricots and raw almonds

Lunch:
Tabouli or other grain-based salad with chopped tomatoes and crumbled goat cheese

Snack:
Celery with peanut butter spread and raisins on top (my daughter's favorite!)

Dinner:
Roasted lamb chops, cucumber salad made with Greek yogurt and mint, sautéed zucchini, red wine (optional)

FRIDAY

Breakfast:
Greek yogurt layered with berries and pumpkin seeds, green tea

Snack:
Poached shrimp wrapped in lettuce leaves

Lunch:
Lentil soup, small green salad with olive-oil vinaigrette

Snack:
Leftover cucumber salad

Dinner:
Roast chicken (don't eat the skin), steamed broccoli, mashed sweet potatoes

SATURDAY

Breakfast:
Orange and grapefruit slices over whole-grain pancakes or waffles, turkey bacon, green tea

Snack:
Edamame

Lunch:
Salad with leftover roast chicken, olive-oil vinaigrette

Snack:
Greek yogurt with blueberries and walnuts

Dinner:
Whole-grain pizza with lots of sauce and veggies, light on the cheese, green salad with olive-oil vinaigrette

SUNDAY

Breakfast:
Scrambled eggs with sautéed spinach, mushrooms, roasted red peppers, chopped tomatoes, and low-fat Swiss cheese, all-fruit smoothie made with half a banana, a handful of blueberries, crushed ice, and a splash of water or coconut water

Snack:
Banana slices with chopped almonds and cinnamon

Lunch:
Turkey chili with black beans and lots of veggies

Snack:
Tofu slice fried in olive oil on whole-grain toast

Dinner:
Halibut, cod, or other fish, seaweed salad with rice wine vinegar and sesame oil, brown rice (my dad's favorite dinner combination!)

6 | IMPROVING YOUR PORTRAIT

Your face is what the world sees first, and people today have become very good at taking exactly the kinds of photos of themselves they want the world to see. The selfie is an interesting phenomenon, because it has taught many people at exactly what angle to hold the camera (slightly above the face), what angle to hold the face (tilted slightly up) and body (at an angle, to minimize width), and what expressions (Duck lips? Wry smiles? Just enough teeth but not too much?) to make for the best possible result. The good ones— the photos where we all look the best—go on Facebook or Instagram or into the family album. The bad ones: delete!

However, camera tricks can go only so far. There is a lot more you can do to get photo ready by improving the look of the parts of you that most often end up in a portrait: the face, neck, and upper chest. These are the areas most subject to sun damage and aging, but there is a lot you can do to keep your portrait features looking younger, smoother, tighter, and more lifted. Let's optimize your future selfies!

LOOSE SKIN

It's a sad fact of life: As we age, skin sags. It happens to everyone, without regard to gender, skin color, or lifestyle. Eventually, your skin will get looser, and that will make you look older. Cheeks sag, necks droop, jowls form, and the skin around your mouth develops deep creases and begins to droop more and more into a natural frown.

For an unlucky few, these changes happen earlier, in the fourth decade of life. For most, the fifties is when these issues really start to become obvious. Virtually everyone in their sixties has some degree of drooping skin and jowl action going on. No matter your age, if you are noticing signs of aging, I know you don't feel ready to look old in those photos. Don't despair—you can turn back the clock! There are many ways to improve the situation, and although surgery is one of them, there are much less invasive and less expensive options, too. Let's look at them.

But first, I have to be straight with you. For many people, plastic surgery isn't an option, and the many strategies I've already talked about are as far as they want to go. However, although this is a book about how to look younger *without* plastic surgery, the simple truth is that the most dramatic and effective way to combat saggy skin really is a facelift. I'm not telling you to get one—most people won't—but I will tell you what's involved so you can decide for yourself.

The Facelift

What exactly is a facelift, and what does it do? Well, before we get into that, let's first describe some basic anatomy. Plastic surgeons divide the face into thirds. The upper third of the face includes the eyes, eyebrows, forehead, and hairline. This area is typically treated with upper eyelid lifts (upper blepharoplasty) and brow lifts. (I'll tell you more about those in chapter 7.) The middle third of the face includes the cheeks and lower eyelids. These areas are treated surgically by lower eyelid lifts (lower blepharoplasty) and cheek lifts (also called mid facelifts). The lower third of the face extends from the cheek hollows downward, including the upper neck and jowls. A facelift typically treats only the lower third of the face. For this reason, a more accurate term for a facelift is a *lower face and upper neck lift*. In my office we shorten it to *lower facelift*, but other offices simply use the term *facelift*.

I tell you all this to explain that a facelift does not treat the upper face. That would be a brow lift. It doesn't lift the cheeks. That would be a mid facelift. Now that we have that out of the way, let's look at exactly what a lower facelift (or just plain facelift) really does.

Plastic surgeons perform a wide variety of facelifts and give them all sorts of different names, like the **Extended SMAS Facelift**, the **MACS Lift**, the **Deep Plane Lift**, and many others. No matter what a facelift is called, they all pretty much work the same way by doing three things:

1. *Removing excess skin.* As your skin loosens and sags with age, a facelift removes some of the excess using incisions (and creating scars) around the ears.

2. *Removing or repositioning excess fat.* As we age, we all develop jowls and excess fat below the jawline. All facelifts either remove this fat or move it up to a higher spot on your face.

3. *Tightening or removing loose muscle.* A thin, sheetlike muscle underlies the skin. In the neck it is called the platysma, and in the face it is called the SMAS.

For those who have a sagging jawline and/or neck and want a dramatic, permanent solution, there simply is no substitute for a facelift. However, a facelift is quite an invasive surgery. It can take anywhere from two to six hours, depending on the surgeon and the technique used. Facelifts create permanent scars around the ears, and recovery time can also be significant, ranging from several days for a mini facelift to several weeks for a more aggressive, deep plane facelift. In general, the more aggressive the facelift, the more dramatic the results, but also the higher the risk of potential complications, such as permanent numbness and facial muscle paralysis, and the longer the recovery time. Obviously, facelifts are not for everyone, but they do get the job done.

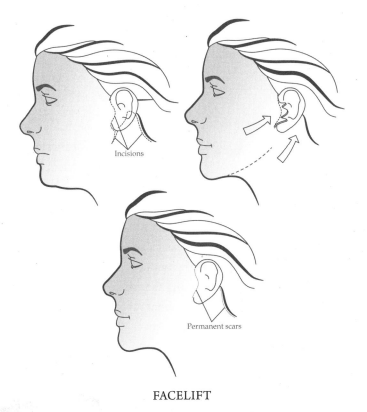

FACELIFT

However, if a facelift is not in your future, there are other options. They may not be as dramatic, but they definitely can be effective and can make a noticeable difference in the sag you don't want to see in those photos of yourself. Let's start with what a doctor can do in the office.

Insider Tip

How do celebs like Barbara Walters, Jaclyn Smith, and Jane Fonda look so good at their advanced ages? Although Jane is the only one of the three who has admitted to having a facelift, I suspect that the other two have had their faces lifted as well. I can't prove it, of course, and would never swear to it in court, but look at their necks. A sharp neckline with no drooping under the chin in a person who's over fifty-five is the best giveaway of a great facelift. Most people over fifty have at least some loose skin on their faces and necks. The other way to tell that someone has had a facelift is to look for the scars in front of the ears. Today's HDTVs often give these scars away.

Ultrasound and Radiofrequency

Laser and other device companies are working feverishly to develop technology that can lift the face without surgery. So far, I've seen some pretty impressive results. Not surgical-quality results, but impressive nevertheless. Typically there are two kinds of devices currently used for nonsurgical facelifts: ultrasound and radiofrequency.

* **Ulthera:** This device uses ultrasound waves to heat up the deeper layers of skin, tightening it. Some doctors have gotten great results with this device, but the treatments can be painful. As of this writing, the Ulthera is probably the gold standard for nonsurgical skin tightening. However, even though it's probably the most aggressive treatment out there, I've seen variable results. I've seen some patients with visibly tightened and lifted skin, and other patients who've paid thousands of dollars to have the procedure, only to see no visible results several months later. If you are considering having this treatment, talk at length with the plastic surgeon or dermatologist administering it to make sure you have a plan in case you don't get the results you are looking for. According to RealSelf.com, a prominent plastic surgery website that allows users to rate and comment on the procedures they've had done, the average cost of Ulthera treatments is $2,675. That's a lot of money to spend on something that could have dramatic results, but which could also have results that are merely minimal.

* **ReFirme:** This device uses radiofrequency waves to tighten up the deeper skin layers. The results are subtle, and the treatment must be repeated for optimal results, but the procedure is virtually painless. Because ReFirme is less aggressive than Ulthera, it costs quite a bit less, averaging $575 according to RealSelf.com. The results, though, in general are more subtle than with Ulthera. There are several other radiofrequency skin-tightening treatments available from other device manufacturers, such as **Pelleve**, **Exilis**, **Fractora Firm**, and **Venus Legacy**. Like ReFirme, these mild radiofrequency treatments require several sessions for optimal results.

Beauty Secret

For an instant jawline lift, contour your neck with a powder that is a shade or two darker than the skin of your face. Start at your chin and work it along your jawline to hide the jowls and make your jawline more defined. Use a blender brush (the kind with a sponge tip) to blend the colors so it's not too obvious, and blend it almost to your ears. Once you are happy with the results, set them with powder.

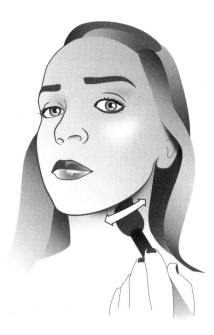

Step 1.   Use color a shade or two darker than the skin of your face and blend under your jawline.

Step 2.   Apply powder to set.

MAKEUP TO CONTOUR JAWLINE

Facelift Creams

If you would rather treat your sagging skin at home, there are some products that give you a pretty good bang for your buck. "Instant facelift" creams are probably the most popular, and there are several available on the market. These work because when you apply them to the skin, you are covering your skin with a thin film that tightens the skin temporarily by causing it to shrink slightly. If you've ever let a few drops of glue dry on your skin, you know the feeling.

One of the most popular instant facelift creams is the **Athena 7 Minute Lift**. This is a quick-lifting cream that includes twelve organic essential oils so your skin gets not just tighter but visibly smoother. Like some of the other instant tightening creams, this one can leave a visible film on the skin if too much is applied. A tiny amount of the Athena 7 Minute Lift goes a long way. If you try it, make sure to play with it, applying it a few times, in order to optimally tailor the application to your skin and create the results that you are looking for. There is definitely a learning curve involved, but the results can be pretty impressive.

The **Epicuren Instantlift Facial Cream** is made by an environmentally conscious skin-care company, and it contains oat and seaweed extracts that combine to immediately but subtly tighten the skin of the face and neck. Like the Athena 7 Minute Lift, the Epicuren Instantlift Facial Cream creates a temporary tightening of the skin, but it can also leave behind a visible film, so be warned. Also keep in mind that once it wears off, your skin won't be improved and it won't look any younger.

Because the results of these kinds of products are temporary, I recommend using them right before a big event, such as before a party, a reunion, or a date, where you want to look as good as possible. By the time the treatment wears off, the party photos will be on Facebook or your date will be long gone, and he or she will be none the wiser! If you use these instant lifters, then be sure to combine them with the long-term use of an antiaging cream like tretinoin (Retin-A). That way, you can get both instant and long-lasting benefits.

DIY Skin Tighteners

If you prefer the all-natural approach, I have another good recipe for you. This homemade scrub will tighten your skin for several hours, so as with the facelift creams, I recommend using this scrub before a big event when you want to look your best. This recipe combines coffee grounds and olive oil. Coffee grounds are full of caffeine, which functions to tighten the skin and can also exfoliate it. Olive oil is full of antioxidants, which neutralize the free radicals that cause skin aging, and also acts as a nice moisturizer. Here's how to make it and use it.

Coffee Ground and Olive Oil Scrub

3 tablespoons coffee grounds

2 tablespoons olive oil

Mix the coffee grounds and olive oil together to create a thick paste. Scrub the paste onto your skin for one to two minutes, then allow to sit for at least five minutes. This is a pretty messy one, and you may find it easier if someone applies it to your face for you. Gently wash the paste off with warm water. Your skin will feel silky smooth for several hours afterward.

Beauty Secret

Makeup won't actually lift your skin, but it can create the illusion of lift. One good way to do this is with blush, which can mimic a cheek lift pretty well. Here is how to apply it:

✳ First, choose the right color. For the best lifting effect, choose a warm-toned blush color. For light skin, choose a shade of pink or apricot. For darker skin, try brown, orange, or burgundy.

✳ Start applying the blush a centimeter or two below the middle of your lower eyelid and extend the blush over the tops of your cheeks, staying in the upper third of your cheek. This causes the cheeks to look higher, as if they've been lifted.

✳ To emphasize the cheek lift even more, apply a darker shadow to the cheek hollows, underneath the apples of the cheeks. You can suck in your cheeks to find where your natural hollows lie. Use an earth-toned shade like brown or taupe, ideally two or three shades darker than your skin tone. Apply with a light hand, and blend well to make it look natural. You don't want stripes!

✳ Once you are happy with the result, set the blush with an overlay of face powder.

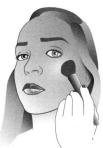

Step 1. Apply blush to the top one-third of the cheek.

Step 2. Apply a darker shadow to the cheek hollows. Suck in your cheeks to find where the natural hollows lie.

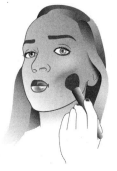

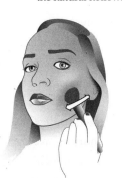

Step 3. Blend it well, then set the brush with face powder.

MAKEUP FOR A CHEEK LIFT

NASOLABIAL FOLDS

These grooves, which extend from the sides
of our noses to the corners of our mouths, are
often referred to as smile lines or laugh lines,
and the deeper they get, the more they seem
to upset the people who have them. How
ironic that the lines from your smile would
make you frown! Yet, nasolabial folds are one
of my most common complaints, right up there
with frown lines, crow's-feet, and saggy necks.

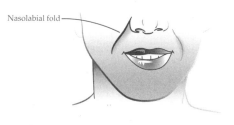

NASOLABIAL FOLDS

Nasolabial folds are actually wrinkles that develop because of the connection
between the skin and the deeper muscles of the face. This skin-muscle connection
functions to hold up the fat of the cheeks. Unfortunately, along with virtually every other
part of our bodies, the fat of our cheeks descends, or sags, as we age. The descent of this
fat over the immobile skin–muscle connection causes the nasolabial folds to deepen.
Basically, the cheek fat droops over the fold. As we get older, these grooves get deeper and
deeper.

Nasolabial folds are static wrinkles because they aren't caused by muscles and are
present at all times. (Dynamic wrinkles are caused by the contraction of muscles under
the skin.) However, smiling and frowning contribute to deepening these creases. But do
you really have to go through life expressionless just to avoid these wrinkles? Of course
not. There is an easy fix, and you may be relieved to hear that it isn't a facelift!

If you've ever stood in front of the mirror and pulled back on your cheeks to make
your nasolabial folds disappear (or at least diminish), then you probably thought
that a facelift—especially a cheek lift—would help these lines look less dramatic.
Unfortunately, this is not the case. Facelifts are great for sagging cheeks and jowls, but
not so great for these smile lines. They really don't do much for them at all. They may look
temporarily better while the face is still tight and swollen immediately after a facelift,
but after just a little bit of relaxation (which occurs with every lifting surgery), and after
the swelling goes down, those pesky lines will return. This was the lesson learned by
the poor guy I told you about at the end of chapter 1 who underwent a quickie facelift in
a misguided attempt to soften his nasolabial folds. In fact, studies have demonstrated
that most facelifts do not improve nasolabial folds.[30] In some cases, when the underlying
muscles of the face are tightened, a facelift could even, theoretically, make these folds
worse. If the folds are really severe, there have been cases when plastic surgeons have cut
the folds out. However, this trades the wrinkles for a scar—something most people aren't

willing to do. This is why most doctors (myself included) almost never recommend a surgical excision of the nasolabial folds. There are much better, quicker, and easier options.

Fillers

The gold standard for treating nasolabial folds is the injection of fillers. This is a procedure you can get in your plastic surgeon's or dermatologist's office. Because these lines are basically just deep grooves in the skin, injecting them with a filler effectively pushes the grooves out, causing the nasolabial folds to become blunted. The key to this procedure is to use enough filler to actually push the wrinkles out. Most fillers are sold in vials of 1 cc each. Some popular brands include **Juvederm** and **Restylane**. One vial will correct only the shallowest of nasolabial folds. If yours are more severe, you will need two or even three vials for full correction. Anything less may be disappointing. The cost per vial ranges from $500 to $900, depending on who's doing the injecting and what part of the face is being injected.

My most common go-to filler for the nasolabial folds is **Juvederm Ultra Plus.** It often lasts longer than the other hyaluronic acid injectables but is slightly softer and easier to inject. I find the results of Juvederm Ultra Plus last between nine and twelve months, sometimes longer. **Restylane Lyft** is a little gritty and has great lifting action but may not last as long as Juvederm. All of these hyaluronic acid fillers are completely reversible with hyaluronidase, if you are unhappy with the results.

Caution!

I have many patients ask me if I can recommend a permanent solution to their nasolabial folds. I strongly discourage any of my patients from having permanent fillers injected into their faces. Permanent fillers, like silicone, can cause permanent problems. There are many things that can go wrong: They can be injected poorly, they can get infected, and the body can create an inflammatory reaction around them. If any of this happens, what is the solution? Unlike hyaluronic acids like Juvederm and Restylane, there is no antidote to them. Unlike with Sculptra or Radiesse, you can't just wait for the product to gradually disappear. The only solution may be to *cut it out of you.* Yes, surgically excise it. Save yourself the potential grief and stay away from permanent fillers!

Facelift Tape

If you don't like the idea of injecting anything into your face and you would rather try something at home, the bad news is that there isn't anything spectacular out there, especially for deep nasolabial folds. However, one temporary solution that may work for you is facelift tape. Facelift tape attaches to your skin or scalp and pulls your skin up. This can improve your nasolabial folds and also lift your jawline and neckline. One popular brand, available online, is **Art Harding's Instant Face Lift**. There is also a product called **Facelift Bungee** that attaches in your hair. I'm not a big fan of these devices, because in general, if someone spots them, it seems to me this could be embarrassing. Although these types of devices may be more visible, they can be valuable ways to test-drive a real procedure to improve your nasolabial folds or lift your face. For that, if for nothing else, I recommend them.

Other than these options, there really isn't any good cream, peel, product, or natural recipe that will make any difference to nasolabial folds. Fillers really are the treatment of choice if you absolutely have to get rid of your nasolabial folds. Anything else is probably a waste of time and money.

PERFECTING YOUR NOSE

Now that we've got your face looking tighter and lifted, let's consider your nose. Noses come in many shapes and sizes, of course, and they can all look fantastic, but the simple fact is that as we age, our noses actually get bigger and longer. They can also get pointier and sharper as the skin of the nose thins with age. This can cause the edges of the underlying cartilage to be more visible. For some people, this may actually improve the look of the nose, but for others, it can look harsh or sharp, or just out of proportion.

You probably notice other people's noses. They are, of course, front and center on the face. They are also notoriously criticized. The eyes, the lips, the skin, all get praised for their beauty-enhancing effects, but not the humble nose. When you think about it, are there any celebs who are known for having a really good-looking nose? Do you ever say, "Wow, his nose aged really well," or "Now, that's a handsome nose on an older woman!" Not really. Just think of all the celebrities with bizarre noses everyone notices. From Jimmy Durante to Owen Wilson, Barbra Streisand to Michael Jackson (whose nose made any self-respecting plastic surgeon shudder), Hollywood is full of bulbous, crooked, oversized noses with bumps, bulges, or the blatant effects of botched surgery—and hardly any of them are aging well. A nose that calls too much attention to itself, especially as it changes with age, can definitely detract from other more attractive parts of the face. Would you rather have someone gaze into your eyes or gaze into your nose? That's what I thought.

You can do a lot with makeup to help your nose (see the Beauty Secret box that follows). A solid skin-care routine and the Age-Fix diet can actually (perhaps surprisingly) be nose friendly as you age. Inflammation exaggerates the aging effects of the nose, especially in people with rosacea or other inflammatory skin conditions. These can add redness and even, eventually, excess tissue to the nose, but the right products (as recommended in chapter 4) and an antioxidant-rich diet may combat this effect.

However, if your nose issues are—in your opinion—more extreme, you have two options: fillers and surgery.

Beauty Secret

Applying makeup in just the right way can make your nose look more like it did when you were younger. This can also slim a wide nose. Here's how:

✳ First, apply a highlighter that is similar in shade to your normal skin color, or possibly slightly lighter, vertically along the center of the nose to increase its projection.

✳ Next, apply a bronzer that is two shades darker than your normal skin with a brush along the sides of your nose. Apply it in an up-and-down motion to create the appearance of shadowing.

✳ Gently blend it in with your fingers or a brush, then apply powder to set the whole thing.

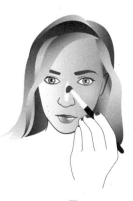

Step 1. Apply highlighter vertically along the center of the nose.

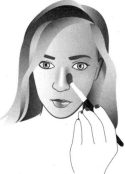

Step 2. Apply a bronzer two shades darker than your normal skin color along the sides of your nose.

Step 3. Gently blend and apply powder to set.

THIN A NOSE WITH MAKEUP

Fillers

More and more plastic surgeons are injecting fillers into the nose to reshape it, which can be a much less invasive option than surgery, even if it is temporary. Especially in people who have a scoop in their noses, injections of fillers like Restylane are viable ways to nonsurgically change the shape of the nose. The procedure is quick and relatively painless (if the doctor uses a numbing gel) and has no downtime. The only drawback is the temporary nature of the results, which typically last for six to twelve months, and the tiny yet significant risk of complications. The risk of injecting the filler into an artery is very small, but slightly higher with nose injections than with those in the nasolabial folds or smile lines. Injecting filler into an artery could result in major complications, such as permanent scarring and worse. Still, if your doctor can reshape your nose with filler and make you happy, then it is certainly a very valid alternative to surgery.

Caution!

The injection of fillers into the nose is considered off-label by the FDA. This is perfectly legal, and it doesn't mean the procedure is unsafe. It only means that the FDA has approved the treatment, but for something different from how it is being used by the physician or surgeon.

Rhinoplasty

If fillers aren't enough to solve your issue, you may already be considering surgery—many people consider a nose job, even if they never get one. Before you make your appointment, consider that many people live with imperfect noses and it doesn't bother them at all (or not much). Also consider whether your nose gives you a uniqueness and character that you love more than you dislike your nose's imperfections. You don't want to be "Jennifer Greyed" with your nose job. Jennifer Grey, you may remember, was America's darling after starring as Baby in the hit movie *Dirty Dancing*. Everyone loved her. I loved her. Several years later she had the bump on her nose removed, and although she looked gorgeous, most people couldn't recognize her anymore. Her acting career quickly declined afterward, perhaps as a result of this change, even though she and her nose looked great.

However, if you are undeterred, and you feel that your nose needs more help than you can provide for it with makeup, products, and diet, then you should know what you are in for with a nose job.

Nose jobs, which are technically called rhinoplasties, are some of the most difficult cosmetic surgeries we perform. A rhinoplasty must be done so precisely (studies show) that even one millimeter of a bump left on the nose could be visible at a normal conversational distance. A rhinoplasty is also extremely complex, because one small change to the nasal cartilage can have several, sometimes unexpected, outcomes in the resulting shape of the nose (as you may have seen with certain celebrities).

Before undergoing rhinoplasty, I advise a realistic self-appraisal (or maybe even a professional one): Do you have a real, bona fide issue with your nose that is worth going under the knife for? Surgery for a bump on the nose or a nose that is becoming longer and sharper with age can make a big difference in appearance, even out of proportion to what you might guess. It can definitely make you look younger. However, it is a surgery not without risks. Because nose jobs are such difficult operations, and each plastic surgeon creates his or her own style of nose, it's best to consult with at least two or three plastic surgeons before settling on one. Make sure you and your doctor are on the same page about the kind of results you want. Sign up for the surgery only when you are convinced that your surgeon understands and is capable of providing you with those results. Also make sure to take a look at your surgeon's "before" and "after" photos to ensure that you like his or her results. If you can't find a plastic surgeon who is on the same page as you, then do not have surgery. That may be a sign that a rhinoplasty may not be in your best interests.

REFINING YOUR LIPS

Who doesn't want a kissable pucker? Mouths, like noses, come in many different shapes and colors as well as shades, but they are not only more of an area of focus (it's where all our words come out!) but sadly much more prone to the effects of aging.

A young-looking mouth can do a lot to make the whole face look younger, and one of the most obvious signs of aging is thinning of the lips. Young people tend to have plump, full lips. Think of Scarlett Johansson, Angelina Jolie, or Brigitte Bardot for those of you from the previous generation. Thin lips are associated more with older people, like Aunt May in the Spider-Man comic books. Of course, not everyone has plump lips, even when young—some people's lips are just naturally thin—but everyone's lips lose volume over time, and plumping up your lips really can erase some years.

The lips are the softest tissue in the body, so any treatment that enhances them must keep them feeling soft and plush. Do you want the person kissing you to feel as if he or she is kissing an old spare tire? No, you want your lips to feel like lips—soft, kissable lips—so keep that in mind. This is one reason I'm not a fan of lip surgery.

Yes, there is such a thing as lip surgery. Surgeons have implanted Gore-Tex into lips as a permanent lip filler, which can create an overly stiff look. They've even used cadaver skin—talk about the ick factor!—which has short-lasting results. Today fat injections are more common, but they give you only a modest, long-term enhancement. So don't bother with the knife to plump up your lips. Try these techniques instead.

Fillers

You're going to think I'm a big fan of fillers, and you would be right. Injectable fillers are the most common way to plump up the lips. I like to describe injectable fillers as liquid skin. We can inject the filler into the borders of the lips to plump them up temporarily. The first commonly injected filler was collagen. Collagen worked well, but it didn't last very long. In fact, most of the time it lasted for only two to four months.

Today, the most popular injectable fillers are made of hyaluronic acid. I've already told you about hyaluronic acid as well as some of these fillers, like Restylane and Juvederm. In these, the injectable filler is in gel form and lasts six to twelve months in most people. If you don't like the results, there is also an antidote: the doctor can inject hyaluronidase to almost instantly dissolve the hyaluronic acid gel. That's important if you develop a complication, such as the accidental injection of the filler into an artery.

You may wonder why, if injectable fillers are so soft and natural these days, so many Hollywood stars have lips that look so unnatural. Maybe you've heard the terms *trout pout* and *fish lips*. The most common reason this happens is because of the alteration of the lip's natural proportions. Normally, the lower lip is 50 percent thicker than the upper lip, but for some reason, many patients insist that they want their upper lips larger than their lower lips. This reversal of the natural lip proportions causes the person to look like a fish—or a duck. For best results, ask your doctor to maintain the natural lip proportions, and your fillers should come out looking much more natural.

Beauty Secret

Not a fan of needles? You can create the illusion of fuller lips through the magic of cosmetics. Here are a few tricks:

* Pretreat the skin just above your upper lip with foundation to prevent your lip color from bleeding into any vertical upper lip lines.

* Use a nude lip liner that's the same color or shade as your lips and apply it around the periphery of your lips. This can define them and make them look slightly plumper. Feel free to experiment with applying the lip liner a little outside your natural lip line, and apply it to make your lips slightly rounder, not straight

across. This can make your lips look fuller, yet they'll still look natural if it's not overdone. (In general, it's good to avoid using lip liner to make the Cupid's bow of your lips look fuller, as this can look fake.)

✳ Apply a medium but somewhat bright shade of lipstick to fill in the newly larger-looking lips. This can make you look younger and more striking. Blot with a tissue, reapply, then blot again.

✳ Finish by applying dabs of nude, shimmery lip gloss on the lips, focusing on the middle of your lips. The shine gives the illusion that they are plumper. Alternatively, you can apply highlighter to the top of your Cupid's bow to make your lips look plumper. Use a shade that is very similar to the color of your lips, and apply in light dabs, such as with your index finger.

Step 1. Apply lip liner a little outside your natural lip line.

Step 2. Fill lips with lipstick, blot, then reapply.

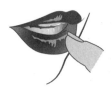

Step 3. Dab with gloss.

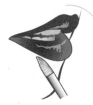

Step 4. Conceal around lips if needed.

PLUMP LIPS WITH MAKEUP

Lip Plumpers

If you would rather plump your own lips at home, there are some effective if temporary topical lip plumpers on the market. Many of them are packaged as combination lip plumpers / lip gloss. Lip plumpers work in one of two ways:

1. One type of lip plumper causes the lips to swell by irritating them, using a substance like peppers, cinnamon, or menthol. These can cause a tingling or even a burning sensation on your lips. You can buy these over the counter, or you can even make your own with this recipe:

DIY Cayenne Pepper Lip Plumper

In a small bowl, combine a teaspoon of petroleum jelly with one drop of peppermint extract and about ⅛ teaspoon of cayenne pepper. Mix it all together, then apply in a very thin film over your lips. If it burns too much, wipe it off and mix in more petroleum jelly to dilute the cayenne pepper. Experiment to get a proportion that works for you. This treatment works and costs just pennies, but it does create a burning sensation, so if you don't like that, see step 2.

2. The other type of lip plumper works by aggressively moisturizing the lips. My favorite product that works this way is **Sexy Mother Pucker Lip Plumping Gloss**. This product is full of volumizing ingredients that help the lips absorb moisture without swelling or pain. It's like filling a raisin back up with juice so it looks like a grape again. This product costs only about $15.

Beauty Secret

If your lips are looking dry and thin and you need a quick fix, try this lip rejuvenation trick: Apply a heavy coating of Vaseline petroleum jelly on your lips and let it sit for ten minutes. Then, with a very soft toothbrush, brush your lips gently to exfoliate the skin. Stop before your lips get irritated or uncomfortable. Follow this up with a good lip balm containing beeswax, such as **Burt's Bees**, or with a combination lip plumper and gloss such as **Bliss Fabulips Instant Lip Plumper**. This treatment not only rejuvenates lips but also can help to reduce those dreaded little vertical lip lines that can form with age and dryness over the top lip. For even better lip line control, apply your regular moisturizer to the skin above the lips to plump it, then apply foundation over the moisturizer to keep gloss or lipstick from bleeding up into the lines. Finish with lip balm containing beeswax or with the Bliss Lip Plumper.

EAR THIS

How bad can your ears be? Nobody really notices them, right? Actually, if you have a torn earlobe, then you might be quite self-conscious about your ears. Earlobe tears are actually fairly common. Heavy hoop earrings may look good, but they wreak havoc on your earlobes, stretching them and making them more susceptible to tearing. Plus, like the rest of our bodies, our earlobes droop as we get older. Unlike the rest of the ear, which is composed of strong, stretch-resistant cartilage, the earlobe is just skin and fat. That means accidents can happen.

Oversized, Stretched, or Torn Earlobes

Earlobes can actually grow with age, and the skin of the earlobes can get droopy, wrinkled, and stretched. Heavy earrings only exacerbate this effect. The piercing in the ear can also stretch. I've talked to some women whose piercing was so stretched that they lost stud earrings when they slipped right through. A more recent trend has made this issue even more common: Young people are wearing earrings of increasingly large gauges, purposefully stretching out their earlobes, often to massive proportions. When the gauge earring comes out, it leaves a droopy, sad-looking lobe that resembles a looped spaghetti noodle. Imagine how these kids' ears will look when they're in their eighties!

It may not surprise you to learn that the only way to permanently fix a torn, stretched, or gauged earlobe is by surgery. The good thing about this surgery is that it is typically performed under a local anesthetic in the office, so there is very little pain associated with it. This is hardly even surgery, unless you consider getting your ear pierced to be surgery. In fact, the procedure can be so quick that I actually performed an earlobe repair on the *Rachael Ray* show while the cameras were rolling!

When the earlobe is torn, the pierced area is typically sutured back together, leaving a small scar. I recommend to my patients to avoid repiercing the ear for at least six weeks, and then have the piercing put in next to rather than in the scar. Even if the scar is completely healed, studies indicate that scarred skin is only about 80 percent as strong as unscarred skin, so if you repierce the actual scar, you are more likely to suffer another tear than you would if piercing in a new location.

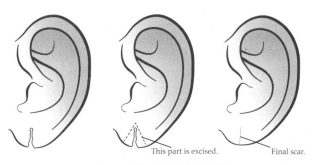

This part is excised.   Final scar.

TORN EARLOBE REPAIR

In the case of an elongated earlobe, the best surgical approach is to cut out a portion of the earlobe. This is also a very simple, quick procedure. The technique I prefer is what I call the **Pac-Man Earlobe Repair**. This entails snipping a pie-shaped portion of excess earlobe out, leaving the earlobe looking like a Pac-Man (if you never played this video game, forgive the reference!). The remaining skin is then sutured back together, leaving the earlobe

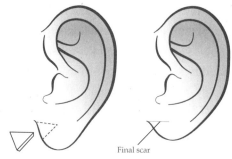

EARLOBE REDUCTION

smaller but with a scar. Another technique involves removing the outer rim of the earlobe, but I've found that it can sometimes leave the earlobe rim looking a bit uneven and unnatural.

Gauge earring deformities can be repaired in a manner similar to that for the elongated earlobe, but it takes more time to make sure the earlobe looks natural. Simply stitching the stretched-out hole together would leave a strangely shaped earlobe, so this takes a little more skill.

Although there is no permanent nonsurgical solution to a torn or stretched earlobe, there are some commercially available patches that fit on the back of the earlobe to temporarily support a torn or stretched earlobe and earring. I like **Lobe Wonder**, which can be purchased online. This small, nearly invisible patch is placed on the back of an earlobe to add support to the earlobe and prevent a stud earring from falling through a piercing. It also decreases the stretched-out look of an elongated earlobe. If you have a cosmetic earlobe problem and don't want surgery, then this could be a good solution for you.

PERMANENT FROWN (AKA "BITCHY RESTING FACE")

Some people's faces naturally form in a permanent frown when they are at rest. We've all seen these people. There was a viral video that described this problem perfectly: "Bitchy Resting Face." The video was meant to be funny, but it was based on a real phenomenon. When certain people's faces are at rest, without making any purposeful expression, their mouths are shaped in a frown, with the corners turned down.

Unfortunately, "Bitchy Resting Face" runs in my family. My paternal grandfather has a permanent frown. My dad has it. I even have a little of it going on. Traditionally, Korean men don't tend to smile in photographs. So when my family gets together for a group photograph, it looks like all the men are angry!

Obviously there is nothing wrong with having a mouth shaped with the corners turning down instead of up, and I would never suggest that anybody who doesn't feel like smiling should try to smile. However, if you have a permanent frown and it really bothers you, you may notice that time just makes it worse. Gravity combined with genetics causes some mouths to head farther and farther south at the corners, giving those people a drooping, grumpy look.

In some people, the problem is compounded by deep grooves on either side of the chin that are appropriately called marionette lines. These really bother some people, and I've even had patients tell me that they develop skin infections and irritations in these grooves. One patient complained that large amounts of food kept getting stuck in them! She would go out to dinner with her friends then come home and look in the mirror at a horrifying sight—poppy seeds and salad dressing stuck in the grooves around her mouth! So what do you do with a permanent frown that has got you down? Turn it around!

Fillers

For most people who would like to lift their permanent frowns a bit, filler injections are the answer. Just as these can help with nasolabial folds, filler injections can also help to lift a frown and to fill in marionette lines. The same fillers I mentioned earlier in this chapter for nasolabial folds are the ones commonly used to treat permanent frowns. They are injected with a small needle, and they typically require no downtime and cause very little bruising. Most people need only one vial to reverse a frown, and the filler can last six to twelve months, occasionally longer.

Botox injections can also be an effective treatment for permanent frowns when they are caused by muscles that actively pull down the corners of the mouth. The plastic surgeon can inject the Botox into certain muscles in the chin that are pulling down the corners of the mouth, and this can give a slight lifting effect. The results last about three to four months, after which you will begin to frown again. Because these results are much shorter than those for fillers, I prefer starting with the filler injections for this issue. Also, if too much Botox is injected, or it migrates, then you could end up weakening muscles that you don't want to. This could leave you looking asymmetric, could prevent you from pursing your lips (no kissing for you!), or, worst of all, could make you look like you've had a stroke.

Grin Lift

You probably don't need surgery for your bitchy resting face. Why not just embrace it? I recently saw an online joke showing a picture of Vivien Leigh as Scarlett O'Hara, with a deadpan look on her face, that said, "Smiling gives you wrinkles. Resting bitch face keeps you pretty." So there's that! However, if your case is extreme and worsening with age, there is a surgery that addresses the problem. It's called a grin lift or corner mouth lift.

This surgery is very simple and short and can be done in the office. The excess skin weighing down the corners of the mouth is excised. This lets the mouth rise back to a more normal position. However, it has one big downside: scarring. You will end up with a small scar extending upward from each corner of the mouth. If this isn't done very well, you could end up looking a little like Jack Nicholson's Joker character in the old *Batman* movie. These scars can remain visible, especially in younger people, who don't scar as well as older people. Because of this, I rarely recommend this surgery for anyone who is younger than fifty-five or sixty.

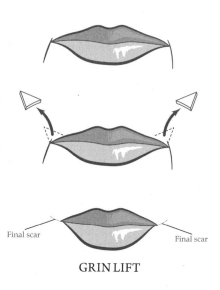

GRIN LIFT

NECK AND DÉCOLLETAGE WRINKLES

I Feel Bad About My Neck. Not only is this a best-selling book by the late Nora Ephron, but it's also a phrase I hear from patients every single day. If your neck concerns involve sagging skin, then take a peek at my recommendations earlier in the chapter for treating the lower face. These suggestions apply to the upper neck as well. If, however, your concerns are wrinkles, then the neck is treated differently than the lower face.

Platysmal Bands

Do you have small bands in your neck that change when you talk, grimace, and make different facial expressions? If so, you have platysmal bands. The platysma, discussed earlier, is the sheetlike muscle of the neck that extends to the lower face. When this muscle stretches with age, it forms these bands that change depending on if the muscle is flexed or relaxed. There is no permanent solution to platysmal bands. Since they are composed of actual muscles, you can't just surgically cut them out. A facelift will improve them, but if you don't want to be that extreme, consider Botox. In cases where the platysmal bands are worsened by excessive contraction of the muscle, injections of small amounts of Botox directly into the muscle can cause it to relax and the platysmal band to smooth out. The effects last for three to four months on average.

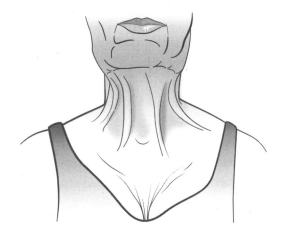

PLATYSMAL BANDS AND
DÉCOLLETAGE WRINKLES

Wrinkled Décolletage

Another frequent area of concern is the décolletage, or the upper chest area around and below the collarbone. This is a common area to show sun damage in the form of wrinkles and crepey-looking skin, and it can definitely make people look older, especially if they diligently treat their faces but forget to treat the area just below.

Fortunately, the same treatments recommended for the face in your daily routine (from chapter 4) can be used as general treatments for the neck and upper chest. Just apply the product all the way down. My go-to recommendation to reverse aging in these areas with commercial skin-care products is to combine a retinol cream with a skin-lightening cream. **Lytera Skin Brightening Complex** by SkinMedica is an all-in-one formula for skin aging that can work well for the chest and neck, since it combines a high concentration of niacinamide to lighten dark spots, retinol to reduce wrinkles and exfoliate and tighten the skin, and antioxidants such as vitamin C to fight off free radicals and prevent future aging. Not only that, but it also comes in a relatively large two-ounce size (compared to many skin-lightening creams, which are sold in amounts half that size), allowing you to cover the large surface areas of your neck and décolletage.

One thing to be aware of: The skin of the neck and chest is typically more sensitive to creams and treatments than the hardier skin of the face. Our facial skin is acclimated to these treatments, whereas our neck and chest skin are not, since we tend to ignore them. Therefore, I strongly discourage trying prescription-strength tretinoin on the neck or décolletage, even if you are tolerating it on your face. Try a milder retinol cream first to make sure you're not too sensitive. Don't forget to apply sunblock as well—the younger you are when you start applying sunblock to your face, neck, and chest, the less damage you will have to undo later.

If you're looking for an instant change in the fine wrinkles of your neck and décolletage, then check out **L'Oréal's Revitalift Miracle Blur**. It's basically a powerful moisturizer with the occlusive dimethicone, which traps moisture in the skin and causes it to look smoother and plumper. Many of the fine lines and wrinkles in the neck and décolletage are caused by skin that has become dry and damaged, so a product like this can provide a wonderful, instant improvement. Feel free to use it on the rest of your face, too, but always combine it with active antiaging products like Lytera for immediate and long-term results.

Beauty Secret

Do you have wrinkles in your cleavage? These are the vertical deep grooves that develop between the breasts in the upper chest caused by a combination of sleeping on your side and aging skin. One way to reduce these wrinkles, or help prevent them in the first place, is to use a special bra that supports the breasts while you sleep on your side. The **Pillow Bra** and the **Breast and Chest Pillow** from Intimia are two options that can be purchased online. Combining a bra like this with the skin creams mentioned above is probably your best, noninvasive way to reduce cleavage wrinkles. It's especially a good idea if you have relatively large breast implants, since they can hasten chest wrinkles.

Are you looking picture perfect yet? Almost, but wait . . . there is one part of your face, a part crucial for a beautiful portrait, that we haven't talked about yet: your eyes. That's because when it comes to antiaging, there is a lot to know about the eyes. So much so, in fact, that they've got their very own chapter. Read on to find out how to maximize the windows to your soul.

7 | EYE REPAIR

When someone looks you in the eye, what do they see? Your soul? Your personality? Or do they see crow's-feet, thin lashes, and drooping lids? Your eyes reveal a lot about who you are and how you live, and both good and poor lifestyle choices—not to mention age—will show up in your eyes. Are they puffy? Underlined with dark circles? Bloodshot? Or are they clear, firm, thick lashed, and sparkling?

We all want beautiful eyes, but if something is detracting from the windows to *your* soul, I can help you throw open the blinds and let your light shine through. Both men and women say that the eyes are one of the first things that attract them to someone. Shouldn't you maximize yours?

THE EYES HAVE IT

Your eyelids contain some of the thinnest, most fragile skin on your entire body. Because of this, eyelid skin will not tolerate the abuse that other skin might, even skin that is mere millimeters away on your face. Although your eyelid skin has probably already sustained some damage (aging, sun, rough handling), it's never too late to start handling your eyes with a more delicate touch and making lifestyle choices that enhance your eyes. Here are a few simple tips to keeping your eyelids (both upper and lower) healthy and youthful:

* **Keep your eyes clean.** Probably the most important thing you can do to keep your eyes looking younger is to gently and completely wash your makeup off at the end of every day. Like the rest of the skin of your face, your eyelids need to breathe

and have the day's worth of pollutants and toxins removed from their surface. Use a gentle cleanser to do this, along with a soft washcloth. If you wake up the next morning with mascara stains on your pillow, you haven't done a good enough job. Tip: Avoid waterproof mascara and eye shadow, as these can be much more difficult to properly and completely remove from your delicate eyelid skin. The benefit you get if you should happen to get caught in a sudden rainstorm or a tearjerker movie is far outweighed by the damage scrubbing and pulling at sensitive eyelid skin can cause as you try to get the stuff off.

* **Try not to rub your eyes.** This really does damage your eyelid skin over time—chronic aggressive rubbing of the eyelids can cause the skin to stretch and even sag.

* **Get your allergies under control.** Chronic swelling and irritation from allergies can wreak havoc on your eyelids, even if you aren't rubbing your eyes. Talk with your physician or allergist about the best ways to keep your allergies at bay and your eyes from being itchy and irritated.

* **Avoid high-salt foods.** Water retention related to high salt intake can worsen eyelid puffiness and even contribute to festoons (this is the name for puffy bags of swelling under the eyes—not nearly as fun as they sound!). Meals from Chinese restaurants, Mexican restaurants, and American chain family restaurants (like Chili's and Applebee's) as well as any fast-food restaurants are the worst. They are loaded with sodium.

* **Get plenty of rest.** Fatigue shows up in the eyes first. We've all looked in the mirror the night of or morning after a bender, or just an all-night study session, and been horrified at the appearance of our eyes. Puffy, bloodshot, dark circles—there's a reason why young partying celebrities always seem to be wearing sunglasses when they head home the next morning!

Lifestyle changes go a long way toward enhancing your eyes and heading off the signs of aging, but what about those pesky problems you already have? Let's tackle them, one by one.

CROW'S-FEET

When Mindy, an attractive fifty-year-old woman, came into my office for Botox injections, I asked her what bothered her most about aging. She looked me right in the eye, pointed to her crow's-feet, and screamed, "Ahhhhhh!" I didn't know what to say, so just in case I didn't fully comprehend, she pointed to her crow's-feet again and repeated herself: "Ahhhhhhh!"

I guess she didn't like her crow's-feet.

Crow's-feet are one of the aging issues my patients complain about the most, and they are among the most common and earliest signs of aging on the face. Crow's-feet are the wrinkles that radiate from the outer corners of the eyes. They are sometimes called laugh lines, which is a much nicer name for them. In fact, there was a study in the scientific journal *Plastic and Reconstructive Surgery* that showed that crow's-feet are associated with happiness in women. I think Mark Twain said it best: "Wrinkles should merely indicate where smiles have been." But even though these lines are associated with smiling and happiness, they really do seem to pose a problem for a lot of people.

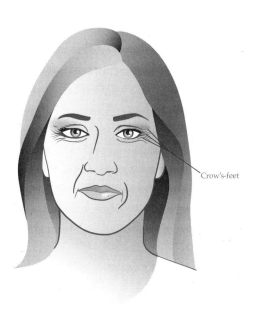

Crow's-feet

Technically, crow's-feet are caused by the action of a circular muscle around the eyes called the orbicularis oculi. These muscle fibers attach to the overlying skin. Years of squinting as well as smiling and laughing create these wrinkles. Fortunately, there are some very effective things you can do to minimize the look of crow's-feet.

CROW'S-FEET

The Gold Standard: Botox

The absolute best way to treat crow's-feet is with Botox injections. This is good news, actually. Botox is much simpler than plastic surgery, and much safer, too. Botox is FDA-approved for treating wrinkles of the glabella and crow's-feet. When Botox is injected into the crow's-feet, it weakens the orbicularis muscles that cause these wrinkles, therefore smoothing everything out. The treatment is extremely easy to perform and takes me about ten to fifteen minutes on average. The effects last for three to four months, and cost varies, averaging $500 per treatment, depending on how much you have done and how much Botox the doctor uses.

Botox injections for crow's-feet rarely have any side effects. Some people may develop a bruise around the injection, but it will fade within a few days. Honestly, there is no better or comparable noninvasive solution for crow's-feet. Botox is the gold standard. It is easy and quick, and for results, nothing comes close. But if Botox really isn't for you, there are other things you can do that will make an impact on crow's-feet, even if it is a lesser impact.

Insider Tip

If you are receiving a Botox injection, make sure your doctor puts his or her finger over the area that is injected and presses down for a few moments. This can limit or prevent bruising. If your doc is in too much of a hurry to do that (for some docs, injecting Botox is like an assembly line: move them in and move them out as quickly as possible), then you can put your finger on the area and press down for a few moments yourself. Then use your other hand to search for a different plastic surgeon or dermatologist in your area.

GABA and DMAE Creams

But maybe Botox still doesn't sound like your thing. Luckily, there are topical solutions that are also quite effective. These creams improve crow's-feet in two ways: by plumping up the skin around the crow's-feet with moisture, or by relaxing the muscles underneath the skin. Creams containing GABA and/or DMAE do the latter by theoretically relaxing the muscles that cause crow's-feet. I say "theoretically," because while GABA and DMAE may be scientifically proven to relax muscles, there is no vigorous scientific evidence that creams containing these products can actually have this effect in real life. That being said, the creams that I've tested do appear to mildly reduce crow's-feet wrinkles. In fact, I tested one cream called the **Nutra-Lift Instant Results Anti-Aging Firming Cream** on national TV and saw an immediate smoothing of the skin that was even visible on camera. I've found some of these creams to be pretty effective for temporary but quick improvement. However, keep in mind that when the cream wears off, you're right back where you started.

If you want to try these creams, look for GABA and/or DMAE as one of the first ingredients listed on the cream. If it's in the middle, or one of the last ingredients on the list, then it's possible the concentration of GABA or DMAE will not be high enough to make a difference.

ZO Hydrafirm

Full disclosure: This eye cream was developed by my good friend Dr. Zein Obagi, a Beverly Hills dermatologist. However, I wouldn't recommend it if I hadn't seen the results myself. It contains a potent combination of vitamin A (similar to tretinoin, which we previously talked about as the number one antiaging skin-care ingredient), caffeine, and shea butter. This is one of the only "instant and long-lasting" age-reducing eye creams that I endorse, and it's an ✳ AGE FIX FAVORITE . The caffeine and shea butter work to instantly smooth and tighten the skin around the eyes, and the vitamin A works to reduce aging long-term on the cellular level. If you were stranded on a deserted island and you could have only one eye cream to bring with you, this would be the one I'd recommend. My patients love it.

Mayonnaise

If you have been waiting for a good natural remedy for crow's-feet, you may be pleased to know that all you have to do is open your refrigerator (or take a quick trip to the market), because mayonnaise isn't just for sandwiches anymore. One of the main ingredients in good old-fashioned mayonnaise is eggs, and the albumin in egg whites is a potent (if temporary) skin tightener. The oil in mayonnaise adds moisture at the same time, making for an effective eye cream. Just apply a small amount of mayonnaise to the crow's-feet area with a cotton ball. Leave in place for approximately thirty minutes, then wash off with warm water and apply your favorite moisturizer. Your crow's-feet will be smoother, and the skin will be much softer and more youthful-looking.

Sweet Potato

Another easy natural crow's-feet treatment is the humble sweet potato. Sweet potatoes are high in vitamin A in the form of beta-carotene, which is a powerful antioxidant and similar to the main ingredient in the classic skin remedies Retin-A and retinol. Sweet potatoes also contain many other vitamins, antioxidants, and minerals that are great for your skin. Try this easy recipe:

Sweet Potato–Yogurt Crow's-Feet Mask

1 sweet potato

4 to 5 tablespoons plain full-fat yogurt

Boil the sweet potato for about thirty minutes (or prick the skin and microwave for ten minutes), cool, then remove the skin. Mash the potato with a potato masher, then mix with 4–5 tablespoons of plain yogurt, depending on how big the potato is. Low-fat yogurt won't work as well as normal yogurt—your skin benefits from the milk fat. The lactic acid in the yogurt also acts as a gentle exfoliator. Combined with the sweet potato, these can reduce wrinkles both immediately and over time. Apply the mixture to your crow's-feet and let it sit for fifteen minutes, then wash off with warm water.

Sunglasses!

I already mentioned the importance of sunglasses in an earlier chapter as a general antiaging (and anticancer) tip, but let me just add that while sunglasses won't fix your crow's-feet and forehead wrinkles, they can definitely keep them from getting worse. The earlier you start, the more prevention you'll be able to effect, because the best way to naturally prevent and treat wrinkles is to quit squinting your eyes. Squinting your eyes causes the orbicularis muscle to adhere more to the overlying skin, making the crow's-feet worse. Sunglasses keep the glare away so you don't have to squint.

Before I had LASIK surgery several years ago, I never wore sunglasses. I had an old pair of prescription sunglasses that grew unfashionable very quickly, so I never wore them. I'd always wear my regular glasses and just squint in the sun. I am convinced that my crow's-feet are worse now than they would have been if I had continued to wear my John Lennon–inspired tinted specs.

DARK CIRCLES UNDER THE EYES

I estimate that at least 75 percent of men and women who see me in consultation for facial aging complain about dark circles under their eyes. These dark circles make them look tired and grumpy, and they can distract people from appreciating a person's other attractive features. But can you really do anything about them, or are you doomed to walk around looking like you've been in a barroom brawl (or haven't slept in a week)?

There is certainly no shortage of creams at the local drugstore or department store that promise to remedy dark circles, but here's the truth: It's all a load of hooey! There are several causes of dark circles under the eyes, and no one cream can remedy all of them. The trick is to get the right product for the right job. For this reason, your first job is to figure out exactly what is causing your dark circles. The treatment will be targeted to the cause.

Dark Circle Culprit #1: Excess Pigmentation

One of my best friends is an Indian woman who has struggled with dark pigment under her eyes for years. She came into my office one day asking for my help on this problem. She'd already tried dozens of creams and none of them helped with her issue. I asked her to bring what she was using, so I could determine whether any of the products would actually help improve the dark pigment under her eyes. She came back with a grocery bag filled with eye creams, from inexpensive grocery store creams to extremely expensive department store treatments. While they all claimed to help dark circles, none of them actually contained any ingredient in a sufficient quantity that would actually lighten skin. What a waste of time and money (and what false advertising!).

People who have darker skin, such as those of Latin, African, Indian, or other Asian origin, are most at risk of pigment-related dark circles under the eyes (you rarely see lighter-skinned folk with dark circles caused purely by pigment). If this is your issue, try these remedies:

* **Hydroquinone:** Creams that contain this ingredient could give you noticeable results within six weeks, but it could take longer if the concentration of the active ingredient isn't very high. Prescription-strength hydroquinone creams are typically 4%, with over-the-counter formulations half that at 2%. If you have easy access to a dermatologist or plastic surgeon who sells 4% hydroquinone products, then go for the higher strength first to see quicker results. Start by using a small amount sparingly, since the undereye skin can be very sensitive.

* **Licorice extract:** If you want to try an all-natural approach, look for creams containing licorice extract. This all-natural skin lightener will probably take longer than hydroquinone to work but is usually well tolerated and can be effective for some people.

* **Niacinamide:** Many over-the-counter eye creams contain this mild skin lightener. Although it takes longer than prescription hydroquinone to work, it's less expensive and easier to obtain. Try eye creams with niacinamide if you are patient and/or on a strict budget. **Olay Regenerist Luminous Dark Circle Correcting Hydraswirl** is one to consider.

* **Retinol eye cream:** Combine one of the above skin-lightening creams with a retinol eye cream for maximal and quickest benefits. Retinol cream can help increase penetration of the lightening agent by causing the upper layer of the skin (the epidermis) to turn over more frequently. Pigmented skin will be sloughed off more quickly. There are several retinol-based eye creams on the market today. I like **Revision Retinol Eye Repair**. ZO Medical's **Hydrafirm** can also be a good option to combine with skin lighteners for dark circles under the eyes.

Dark Circle Culprit #2: Transparent Skin

If your skin is thin and transparent, you could be able to see the dark blood vessels underneath. This is actually quite common in Caucasians. The skin under the eyes is the thinnest skin on the body, sometimes just several cell layers thick. As we get older, the thin eyelid skin gets even thinner. The best way to treat this problem is to thicken that skin.

* **Retinol cream:** Retinol cream is the first thing to try. Not only can retinol cream cause better penetration of lightening creams, but it can also thicken the skin within four to six weeks, causing less transparency and visibility of blood vessels. However, some retinol products are too strong for the delicate undereye area, so make sure the retinol product is formulated specifically for the eye area. Avoid applying prescription-strength tretinoin to your sensitive eyelid skin, as it could cause irritation. A few of the highly regarded brands to look for include **RoC**, **Murad**, and **Dr. Brandt**, or Revision Retinol Eye Repair, mentioned above.

* **Peptides:** If your sensitive undereye skin cannot tolerate retinol, then try using mild peptides, which can also increase the growth of collagen. **D·E·J Eye Cream**, also by Revision, contains a mixture of peptides, antioxidants, and moisturizers to firm and hydrate the skin. Another good option is **DERMAdoctor Wrinkle Revenge Rescue and Protect Eye Balm**, which also uses a combination of peptides, antioxidants, and moisturizers to improve the appearance of the lower eyelids.

* **Moisturizer:** An even simpler solution to transparent skin is hydration, which plumps the skin, decreasing blood vessel visibility. Any eye moisturizer can work for this. There is no problem with this approach, but you won't get any long-term age-reversing effects from it.

Beauty Secret

If you need your dark circles to vanish immediately, makeup can sometimes do the trick pretty well. However, sometimes foundation isn't enough to cover dark undereye circles. If the circles are too dark, then a concealer can make your dark circles disappear. Concealers are similar to foundation but give you more coverage, because they are more opaque. They often come in a tube, a stick, or pancake form. Here's how to use them:

* Choose a creamy concealer in a shade that's as close to your skin tone as possible. Try to resist the impulse to choose a concealer color that is too light–this is a common mistake, and it can make you look like Shamu. Also avoid those concealers that look yellow or even green. Despite what the packaging says, they are likely to just make your skin look yellow or green. Instead, look for more golden tones that match your skin. Try salmon, peach, or light peach if you are Caucasian.

✳ Apply an eye cream first, to moisturize the skin and reduce the appearance of wrinkles. To apply concealer, gently brush or dab with your pinky finger from the inner corner of the eye to the midpoint of the pupil. Feather it out over the rest of the undereye area to blend it in. Don't overuse it–a little concealer goes a long way, and you can always add a little more, but if you overdo it and get a caked-on look, you'll have to wash your face and start over.

✳ Next, apply a light layer of foundation over the concealer. Set the foundation by applying loose translucent powder over the area with a powder puff or powder brush.

✳ If you can still see those dark circles, you can apply a very small amount of concealer on top of the foundation for a final layer of coverage.

Step 1. Apply a moisturizing eye cream.

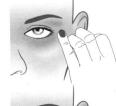

Step 2. Apply a creamy concealer the same color as your skin tone with a brush or your pinky finger.

Step 3. Apply a light layer of foundation over the concealer.

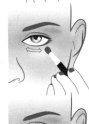

Step 4. Apply powder to set the foundation.

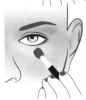

CONCEAL DARK CIRCLES UNDER
YOUR EYES WITH MAKEUP

Dark Circle Culprit #3: Puffiness Causing Shadowing

Probably the majority of complaints I hear about dark circles are related to puffiness, which can create shadowing. This is often caused by fat pockets protruding from your eye sockets. It's a very common condition, virtually universal by the time we enter our sixties.

One way to determine if puffiness is the cause of your dark undereye circles is by seeing if your dark circles are impacted by the level of light. If your dark circles are worse in certain lights, or disappear when you hold your head at certain angles, then it's likely that they are caused by shadowing from the puffiness under your eyes. Quite often, they look much worse in a room with dim lighting. My patients tell me things like, "I was at a party at a friend's house last night and glanced at a mirror and was horrified. My dark circles were worse than ever!" I tell you, I notice this with myself, too. This is because in certain kinds of lighting, the shadows from the puffiness are accentuated.

My office is quite bright, so I often have patients tell me that their undereye circles have mysteriously disappeared when they come to see me. You can also appreciate this on a bright, sunny day. In these conditions there is little shadowing, since the light is bouncing off so many surfaces that people with puffy eyes often find the dark circles look a lot better.

The obvious solution to this sort of shadowing is to get rid of the puffiness. One reason people get puffiness under the eyes is water retention from high salt intake. Allergies and crying can also add to the puffiness. There is also a genetic component. Undereye bags run in families. If you have undereye bags, then it's quite possible your children will have them, too.

So what can you do about these fat pockets, caused by genetics, aging, allergies, or all of these? There are a couple of options.

Surgical treatment: I know this is a book about nonsurgical options, but when it comes to these fat pockets, the only permanent solution is surgery. The surgery can now be done without any visible scars. It is called scarless blepharoplasty. During this procedure, an incision is made on the inside of the eyelid, and the puffy fat is removed, with the scar left on the inside of the eyelid where it cannot be seen. Patients heal very quickly from this surgery, and some have no bruising and very little swelling at all. The limitation of this operation is that excess skin from the eyelids can't be removed. Many people have excessive crepey, wrinkled skin in addition to the excess fat. This surgery doesn't do anything for the excess skin. The operation takes about an hour and has very little pain in the recovery. You may take a pain pill or two, but that's usually it. The cost is typically about $2,500 to $5,000, with the higher end being in bigger cities with big-name plastic surgeons.

If you have both puffiness and excess, crepey skin, then I typically recommend a pinch blepharoplasty, where both puffy fat and crepey skin are removed. The fat is removed via an incision inside the eyelid, like in a scarless blepharoplasty, and the skin is removed by cutting it out from the front of the eyelid. The surgery leaves a tiny, usually imperceptible scar right underneath the eyelashes and costs about the same as a scarless blepharoplasty.

I think both the scarless and the pinch blepharoplasty procedures are quite effective for undereye fat pockets, but there are some surgical techniques that I'm not a big fan of. One is called a fat-repositioning blepharoplasty. Instead of removing the fat from the lower eyelid, some doctors will redistribute it along the tear trough (the groove that extends diagonally down the front of your cheek) or along the crease under your eye along the bone. Ideally this can decrease these grooves, but in worst-case scenarios, it can make the area look lumpy and unnatural.

A canthopexy is a procedure to tighten the lower eyelids when they are loose or droopy, and often to tilt the lower eyelids up, creating more of a cat-eye appearance. It's also similar to the look that resuts when women pull their hair back really tightly and their eyelids tighten and tilt up. In inexperienced hands, this procedure can make you look like a villain from a Disney cartoon. In select cases, however, this procedure can really help people in their sixties and seventies with saggy lower eyelids. I typically refer these types of patients to an oculoplastic surgeon, or an ophthalmologist with specialized training in plastic surgery of the eyelid.

Caution!

Keep in mind that if you have problems with dry eyes and use moisturizing eyedrops, then a lower blepharoplasty (the general name for any kind of blepharoplasty affecting the lower eyelid, both pinch and scarless) may cause your symptoms to worsen. Discuss this with your plastic surgeon and even your ophthalmologist prior to undergoing any surgery to make sure this won't become an issue for you, or to learn what you can do about it if it does become a problem.

Sudden Change Under-Eye Firming Serum: I first discovered this product when a patient came in to consult on a lower blepharoplasty. She said, "I hate the puffiness under my eyes! The only thing that makes it go away is this topical serum I buy at CVS for $12!"

I did a double take and said, "Seriously? You buy an undereye serum at CVS for $12 that makes your undereye puffiness disappear? You're kidding me, right?"

"I'm serious!" she said. "And it works in just three minutes! The puffiness goes away!"

I asked her if she had it with her, and she told me she always carries it in her bag wherever she goes so she can apply it whenever she needs to. I asked her to apply it in front of me and sure enough, after three minutes her undereye bags were *gone*. I was impressed. Since then, I've demonstrated this inexpensive serum on several television programs, always with the same audience reaction: oohs and aahs! It's one of the rare drugstore-bought, inexpensive skin-care products that actually do what they advertise and is therefore an ✺ AGE FIX FAVORITE .

So how does Sudden Change work? Remember how I told you that mayonnaise can help tighten up crow's-feet? Like mayo, Sudden Change contains albumin, which is formulated to provide a shrink-wrapped look under the eye, tightening the droopy skin. Within minutes, the albumin temporarily eradicates undereye bags. You can mix it with your foundation, and although it does not create a permanent change, it's great to use right before a big event like a wedding, a class reunion, or a big date. Just keep in mind that it wears off, so make sure to plan accordingly and keep a container with you to reapply when necessary. Don't apply too much, or it can leave a visible film behind. Experiment before it really matters to see how much is just enough to get a good effect without that filmy residue. Just remember, albumin doesn't take the place of a good antiaging eye cream with retinol and antioxidants. It is purely a quick fix for that special event—and it only costs about twelve bucks! I suspect that Sudden Change is used by more than one celebrity on the red carpet.

Potato and green tea eyelid lift: For a natural and inexpensive approach, try this DIY eyelid lift, which works both immediately and long-term. Just steep one green tea bag in one cup of hot water in the morning, then put the tea in the refrigerator. In the evening when you get home, cut one raw white potato into thin slices and drop the slices into the tea. Put them back in the refrigerator for a few minutes, allowing the green tea to soak into the potato.

Next, apply a potato slice to each eyelid. Relax and let them sit for ten minutes. After you take off the potato, you will notice that the puffiness under your eyes is significantly improved. You will also notice a reduction in wrinkles and tighter skin. This happens because the starch in the potatoes acts as an anti-inflammatory, soothing the irritation from a long day of pollutants, toxins, and stress. The potato starch is also a mild skin lightener, so it can help gradually reduce dark circles under the eyes caused by excess pigmentation over time. Green tea contains caffeine, which acts as a vasoconstrictor. It can immediately reduce swelling and tighten the skin under the eyes, causing a rapid and significant improvement in puffiness. Green tea is also full of antioxidants, which can help combat free-radical damage from the day. Keep the remaining potato slices soaking in the tea in the refrigerator for up to three days and use nightly, or every morning and every night. This is also a good remedy for morning eye puffiness.

DROOPY BROWS

Have you ever noticed that people tend to look grumpier as they age? There are some very specific reasons for this. With age, gravity exacts a few penalties: It pulls the eyebrows down, pulls the cheeks down, and with a lot of squinting and frowning, creates those "11 sign" lines right between the eyebrows and frown lines along the sides of the mouth.

A very common celebrity fix for droopy brows is a surgical brow lift. Lifting the brows alone can do a lot to change this expression of grumpiness. However, the idea of a surgical brow lift makes people nervous. Many of the celebrities whose plastic surgery results are startling and disturbing look that way because of bad brow lifts. This procedure can make people look like they've just seen a ghost! But for every example like this, there are countless other examples of people who've had brow lifts that have made them look incalculably better. One celeb who I believe had a well-performed brow lift is Sharon Osbourne. Her eyebrows look more alert, refreshed, and youthful than they did thirty years ago! Keep in mind that even if brows are surgically elevated, they tend to settle with time.

Brow lifts are fairly extreme surgeries, however, so let's look at the many other options first.

Brow Lifts with Botox

Botox (or one of its neurotoxin competitors, like **Dysport**) can be used to create a modest brow lift. In people who have droopy brows, or brows that are relatively horizontal in shape, Botox can be injected into certain areas to create an arching, or lifting, of the brows. Good plastic surgeons and dermatologists know how this works and should be able to create this without much difficulty. If your eyebrows are already quite arched, this may not be a good procedure for you, however. It can overarch the brow, giving you a wicked Cruella De Vil look. I call this the Botox Brow, and I think I've spotted it on quite a few celebs.

Interestingly, since Botox has hit the cosmetic scene, the number of brow lift surgeries has declined, and it continues to decline year after year. I perform brow lifts only a couple of times per month max, as most people find that Botox works well enough for them. In addition, Botox is a lot cheaper than surgery, costing approximately $300 to $500 to treat the forehead.

Beauty Secret

You can make a big difference in the appearance of your eyes with a good brow-plucking session, but if you are unsure about plucking your brows or new to shaping your eyebrows, I've got some useful tips for you:

* Brow shaping takes practice and can be a precision operation. Ideally, let your brows grow out, then have a professional shape them for you. Or, if you already have very full brows with little shape to them, have a professional shape them for you.

* If you want to do it yourself, get a magnifying mirror and very conservatively pluck hairs that grow out of place, checking back every week or so.

* One way to determine how they will look before you pluck is to use a white pencil to draw over the hairs you plan to remove. If this looks good, go ahead and tweeze the white ones.

* If your skin is sensitive to plucking, try applying a little toothache medicine over the skin to numb it.

* Pull the hairs out in the direction they grow for the least irritation.

* Always pluck hairs on the undersurface of your brow. Remember that plucking the underside lifts brows, while plucking the top lowers brows, making you look grumpy and older.

* Avoid overthinning of your eyebrows. You don't have to look like Brooke Shields in the 1980s, but keeping your brows slightly fuller gives you a younger, more pleasant look. Compare this to the thin, overarched eyebrows of cartoon witches, and you'll see what I mean.

* Try to follow the natural shape of your brows. Don't try to reshape them into something that they aren't. This could end up looking like an unnatural disaster.

* If your eyes are smaller, your brows should be fuller. If your eyes are larger, your brows should be narrower.

* If you've been overplucked and want your eyebrows to be thicker, try to use an eyebrow stencil (don't try freehanding it unless you're a real artist!) and use a color that is a little lighter than your hair. The exception to this is in very light blonds, where the eyebrow would be washed out. Use a color that is two shades darker than your blond hair. Use a freshly sharpened brow pencil. Fill in sparse areas by using light, fine, irregular marks of the pencil.

* Do not use black to fill in the eyebrows. It can look fake and overdone.

* Another way to brighten your look is by tinting your eyebrows a shade or two lighter than their natural color. This can help to open up your eyes and make you look younger. Ask your salon stylist, who can do your eyebrows at the same time she does your hair.

* To thicken your eyebrow hair, try Latisse (see page 136), and apply very accurately and sparingly to areas of hair loss. Make sure that it doesn't drip down your cheek, though.

Ulthera

Another option for lifting the brow is **Ulthera**, which was discussed at length in the last chapter. It's FDA-approved for lifting the brows, and I've seen its results vary from impressive to invisible. It's possible the results can be dependent on who does the procedure, the settings used, and how a person's skin reacts to it. I recommend that you carefully study the "before" and "after" patient photos from the doctor performing the procedure and make a plan with the doctor for what will happen if you don't get the results you are looking for.

OTHER BROW LIFT OPTIONS

The other options you can try at your plastic surgeon's office to lift your brow are a skin-tightening laser or a chemical peel of the forehead. These both tighten the skin, causing the eyebrows to be slightly elevated. However, lasers and peels are really better for smoothing the skin and reducing fine lines than they are for actual lifting, so they aren't my top choice for people with truly droopy brows. These are relatively inexpensive options, however, with no recovery time.

Instant Forehead Smoother

If you would rather try something at home than in a doctor's office, **Instant Forehead Smoother** is a cream that I tested out on a national television program; it promises instant smoothing of the forehead within minutes. I've seen nice results with this cream, where the brows appeared mildly lifted and the forehead wrinkles a bit smoother. The product can be purchased online from Bremenn Labs. Keep in mind that the cream isn't a substitute for some of the antiaging creams I've already mentioned that focus on longer-lasting results. It's an instant-change cream that should be used along with creams that reverse aging long-term, like Retin-A and creams with growth factors and peptides.

Beauty Secret

Cosmetics can do wonders to open up droopy eyes. Try these techniques:

* Apply eyeliner only to your upper eyelids, or only to the outer third of your upper eyelids. End it on a slight upward slant by turning it up at the corner. This creates a lifting effect to the eyes.

* Apply thicker mascara on the outer corners of your eyes. This makes them appear more open and younger.

* Curl your lashes for a significant lifting effect. The best time to curl them is right when you get out of the shower, but after the eyelashes are dry (wet eyelashes don't curl well). The hot water will soften them and make them easier to curl and less prone to breaking. You can also point a warm hair dryer at the curler for fifteen seconds to warm it up first. This can cause the curl to hold better.

* For the lower eyelids, either skip the eye shadow or use one that is several shades lighter than your eyeliner.

Open Brow Lift

Finally, if other options don't work and you are committed to a brow lift, let's talk about what that involves. There are two types of brow lifts: open brow lifts and endoscopic brow lifts. No plastic surgeon would dispute the effectiveness of an open brow lift. It is truly the best way to lift the brows, with the best long-term results. However, the open brow lift has some significant negatives associated with it.

In an open brow lift, the plastic surgeon makes an incision from ear to ear, either across the scalp or along the front of the hairline. He or she then lifts the forehead skin off the forehead bone and pulls it back, cuts off the excess skin, and staples it into place. This pulls the eyebrows up into a higher position, thereby improving the drooping eyebrows. My former mentor in Beverly Hills performed this surgery all the time with great results. However, as you can probably tell from the description, this is a very invasive surgery. Your forehead is literally lifted off your skull and pulled upward. It's a gruesome and bloody operation, too, with staples extending from one ear across the scalp to the other side. The long ear-to-ear scar can be visible in people with short hair, and the surgery comes with a higher risk of a permanent bald area and postoperative numbness.

Another option for an open brow lift is to put the scar along the front of the hairline. Some surgeons claim that patients like it, but I've never seen a scar along the front of the hairline that I've liked. Remember, scars are permanent, and if your hairline recedes, then the scars might become quite visible. With

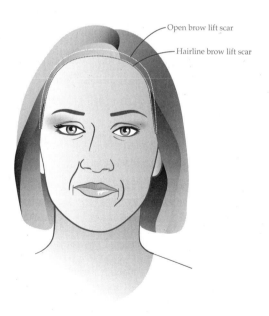

Open brow lift scar

Hairline brow lift scar

BROW LIFT SCARS

the advent of high-definition television, I've been able to spot the telltale hairline scars in several prominent male celebrities. If you look closely, you can probably spot them, too. The hairline looks almost too sculpted, which is a result many people fear when contemplating a brow lift like this.

Because of these issues, I haven't performed an open brow lift in over ten years. Some surgeons are still adamant that this is the way to go, but I think the invasiveness of the procedure outweighs the benefits. Who wants to have their scalp sliced in half if they don't really need to—or even if they do, but only because they want to look a little less grumpy? It seems like an extreme solution to a relatively minor problem. It's also costly—between $4,000 and $7,000.

Endoscopic Brow Lift

In this surgery, the plastic surgeon makes five small incisions in the scalp a few centimeters behind the hairline. Through these incisions, the plastic surgeon uses fiber-optic scopes and instruments to peel the skin off the forehead and pull it upward. Because the skin is pulled off the forehead bone from the inside, there isn't nearly the bleeding that you have with the open approach. The brows are secured in a higher position by placement of either small screws and sutures or an absorbable device called the **Endotine**. It's basically like a carpet tack for the forehead. By the time the Endotine implant dissolves in a couple of months, the forehead has healed into its new, higher location. The surgery also typically costs between $4,000 and $7,000.

This may sound like a preferable option to you, but the problem with the endoscopic brow lift is that I've found the results aren't as predictable as those achieved with an open brow lift. In some patients, the eyebrows tend to settle as it heals, and the eyebrows don't end up quite as high as you would like them to be. Still, it's better than having an ear-to-ear scar and all the potential problems that may come with an open brow lift.

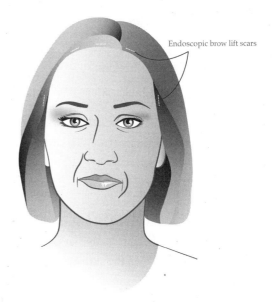

Endoscopic brow lift scars

ENDOSCOPIC BROW LIFT SCARS

Brow lifts are great for a very specific purpose—lifting the brow so you look more alert, awake, and pleasant. But they don't do anything else. They don't remove forehead wrinkles or tighten the skin in any way that makes you look younger. The only way to really effectively reduce forehead wrinkles is with Botox—and Botox is a whole lot cheaper and less invasive.

Insider Tip

Years ago I had a thirty-year-old woman come in to see me in consultation for a brow lift. It took her four years to save $6,000 for the surgery, and she was ready and raring to go. After taking one look at her, I sent her to my aesthetician. Twenty minutes later, her brows were lifted and she paid a grand total of thirty bucks. So what's the secret for a $30 brow lift? Tweeze those brows! If your eyebrows are a tad on the bushy side, you may be able to get a nice brow lift by simply removing the hairs on the undersurface of the brows. This can increase the space between your eyelids and your brows, causing them to look lifted. Note that this works only by removing hairs from below the brow. If you have droopy brows, use caution when removing hair from above the eyebrows, as this can produce the exact opposite effect and cause your brows to look even droopier.

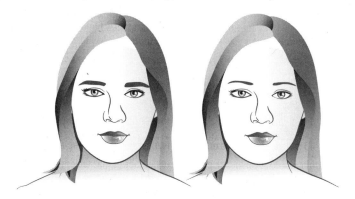

BROW LIFT WITH WAXING OR TWEEZING

DROOPY EYES

The brows aren't the only facial feature that droops. Frankly, your whole face can droop, but drooping eyes are a problem that really bothers a lot of people. As with the rest of our skin, gravity pulls on the skin of our eyelids, causing them to stretch and sag. Sun damage and other environmental insults can make this worse. Sometimes the excess skin is combined with sagging of the brow, making the eyelids look even heavier. When it gets bad, the actual eyelids can become completely covered by skin that has folded over, so you can't see them anymore. This can cause your eyeliner and other makeup to smudge horribly. In the worst cases, it can get so severe that vision is affected. Some people may find that they can't see traffic lights without actually lifting their heads.

Unfortunately, this is one of the few aging issues for which there is no good nonsurgical solution. If this is a problem for you, you may want to consider the surgical options, some of which are very easy and only minimally invasive. Ask your doctor about an upper blepharoplasty, which removes excess skin (and sometimes puffy fat) of the upper eyelids. The surgery typically leaves a small scar in the eyelid crease that is usually well hidden. I call this beginner's facial plastic surgery, because the procedure takes only about an hour and has almost no pain afterward. Most of my patients don't need to take any pain pills. This is one of my favorite procedures to perform, because it can take ten years off a person's appearance in a quick and easy way.

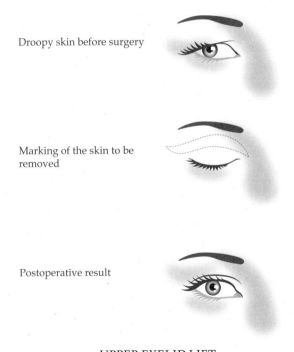

Droopy skin before surgery

Marking of the skin to be removed

Postoperative result

UPPER EYELID LIFT

Unfortunately, like any other cosmetic surgery, it can be overdone. If too much skin is removed, the patient may not be able to close her eyes afterward, leading to issues with dry eyes and even damage to the cornea. An upper blepharoplasty can be a feminizing procedure if overdone, so if you're a man considering this operation, make sure to ask your surgeon to be conservative. You can always take more skin off later if you want, but it's much harder to put it back on once it's removed. Kenny Rogers admitted several years ago to undergoing a botched upper blepharoplasty. One day he showed up on *American Idol* looking strangely feminine. His surgeon apparently removed too much skin. Other celebrities have also appeared suddenly looking quite different after brow lifts (most haven't admitted them, but I have my suspicions). This is just a warning to be very careful with any plastic surgery, especially eyelid surgery. It *will* change how you look, and although in the majority of cases the end result is worth it, for some people surgery can be the wrong choice.

Insider Tip

Insurance companies don't typically pay for plastic surgery if it is for aesthetic reasons only. However, many people don't know that insurance may pay for your eyelid lift. If you have so much skin on your upper eyelids that it impinges on your vision (such as making you miss traffic lights, or if it makes you feel like a window shade is coming down on your vision), then you may qualify for this coverage. Typically, insurance companies require at minimum verification that you are having problems with seeing in the above quadrants of vision by having testing done in an optometrist's or ophthalmologist's office. Most good plastic surgeons are very careful to do a nice, cosmetic job in addition to simply solving the vision problem, so you can get the aesthetic benefits along with the medical coverage.

THIN EYELASHES

Most men don't realize how important eyelashes are to women. Like hair elsewhere, our eyelashes change as we age. They thin, become more sparse in number, and can even become lighter in color. Some people are born with thin eyelashes, and others lose a lot of their eyelashes by overuse or abuse of eyelash extensions and even waterproof mascara.

Fortunately, there are a multitude of treatments to enhance your eyelashes. We'll start with the most extreme and work backward.

Latisse

The gold standard for eyelash enhancement is undoubtedly Latisse. I introduced Latisse to audiences of the *Rachael Ray* show once it hit the market back in 2009. It's been a huge seller ever since and is an ✺ **AGE FIX FAVORITE** . Latisse originated from an antiglaucoma drug called Lumigan, which was produced by Allergan, the makers of Botox and Juvederm. They found that senior citizens taking Lumigan for glaucoma would come back to their ophthalmologists with these gorgeous, full, luscious eyelashes. Knowing a good thing when they saw it, the company created a form for cosmetic use called Latisse and had it approved by the FDA.

It takes about eight to twelve weeks for Latisse to have a noticeable effect, but it is scientifically proven to lengthen, darken, and thicken your eyelashes. Believe me, it works. We've sold many hundreds of boxes of Latisse in my office the last several years, and I've never had a single person return it. In rare cases, it can cause some mild skin irritation, but is otherwise very well tolerated. Reports that Latisse can change the color of your eyes are overblown. This has occurred with Lumigan, but only when it was applied as an eyedrop. It's extremely unlikely for Latisse, when applied as directed on the upper eyelids, to cause this to happen, so if you love your light blue eyes, I wouldn't be too concerned. The main drawback to Latisse is that you must purchase it in a doctor's office. And it's not cheap. A ten-week supply runs approximately $150 to $175. Keep in mind that once you stop applying Latisse, the effects begin to wear off, so you need to use it continually if you want to maintain the good results. As a general rule, it takes as long to wear off as it takes to work—about eight to twelve weeks.

Insider Tips

Insider Tip #1: I get a lot of patients asking me how they can make Latisse more affordable and lengthen the amount of time each bottle of solution lasts them. Well, it's actually pretty easy. The 5 cc box is meant to last approximately ten weeks, and it comes with a total of 140 applicators, so you can use one applicator for each eyelid every day. In this way, after seventy days, you run out of applicators and must buy another box. One simple solution to increase the amount of time your Latisse lasts you is to put a drop on one applicator, and use it on your right eye, then your left. Throw the applicator away. The next day put a drop on a new applicator, then apply to your left eyelid and then your right. Continue on this alternate application path, and your ten-week kit will last you double that!

Insider Tip #2: Are your eyebrows too thin? One great way to make them look thicker is to use a freshly sharpened eyebrow pencil with a stencil. Use a color that is a little lighter than your hair and make fine, feathery, irregular marks to fill in the eyebrows. In the evening, apply a little Latisse to the sparse areas. Most people will see thickening of the hair within two months! Keep in mind that using Latisse for thinning eyebrows is an off-label treatment.

Over-the-Counter Alternatives to Latisse

There are other over-the-counter alternatives to Latisse that are worth checking out if you cannot make your way to a plastic surgeon's office or can't afford it. Obagi Medical Products makes **Elastilash**, which has a different active ingredient that has been deemed effective by scientific studies. You can also check out **RevitaLash** and **Marini Lash**, which can be purchased online or in department stores. I've heard my patients say good things about both of these products.

EYELASH TRANSPLANTS

Believe it or not, some plastic surgeons and hair transplant specialists are actually performing eyelash transplants. For women who have no eyelashes (or a major paucity of lashes), they can take hair from another part of the body and implant it into the lash line of the eyelids. A good friend of mine and prominent hair transplant expert in Florida, Dr. Alan Bauman, performs this procedure.

In the past, the main concern for patients undergoing eyelash transplants was whether the lashes were going to grow in the correct orientation and direction. With the newest techniques, these concerns are no longer problems. There is one caveat to eyelash transplants, however: The new lashes need to be curled and trimmed regularly. Unlike normal eyelashes, the body doesn't have a built-in mechanism to cause them to stop growing once they become a certain length. Transplanted eyelashes just grow and grow and grow. The procedure is fairly unusual, however, and I don't necessarily recommend it. I have never performed it myself.

When your eyes are bright, clear, firm, and fully lashed, you feel beautiful, so don't neglect this most eye-catching part of your face. Whether you choose to make minor changes or major ones, your eyes are worth your attention. Use a gentle hand, and let your natural beauty shine through.

8 | RESHAPING YOUR CURVES

Your face may be the thing people notice the most about you, but you've got a whole lot of body left below the neckline, and many of my patients complain that they have just a little too much here, not quite enough there, and why is it all so much lower than it was a decade ago? Welcome to the aging body, and take heart: There is much we can do to shape it, rearrange it, and keep it looking improbably young.

First and foremost, I would be remiss if I did not remind you of something you probably already know: the number one thing you can do to keep your body looking younger is to exercise regularly. This isn't just a theory or my own crazy idea. There are about a million studies that support this. Exercise actually reverses many of the signs of aging in some pretty dramatic and surprising ways. It triggers chemical processes in the body that build muscle, burn fat, maintain mobility as you age, give the brain an antiaging biochemical bath, and even make the brain bigger![31]

The best effects come from an exercise habit—not exercising once a month, not whenever you remember you have a gym membership, but regularly, as in three to five times per week for at least thirty minutes. This isn't a fitness book, and you can look elsewhere for more information about this, but just know that whether you walk, run, lift weights, do yoga, or do a little of all those things (that's probably the best idea), you will give your entire body, inside and out, a hall pass on aging. You'll still get older, but you won't get older as fast, or look as old as others your age who don't exercise. There was even a study that showed that in mice, regular exercise not only kept organs like the brain and the heart healthier, but actually kept the mice's fur from graying as quickly, and resulted in fewer wrinkles! Follow-up human studies echoed the mouse studies, showing that among those who exercised for three hours every week, skin was thicker, had a more youthful appearance, and even appeared to rejuvenate in older subjects who exercised regularly.[32]

Genetics is another important factor in aging bodies as well as aging faces. Some people have genes that seem to keep them looking and feeling younger, and even shaped like a younger person, all the way into their seventies. Many celebrities come to mind, such as Audrey Hepburn, Jane Seymour, Pierce Brosnan, Denzel Washington, and Michelle Pfeiffer. However, most of the time, for most people, even those who exercise, aging eventually creeps in. Things start to sag. Fat accumulates in places where we don't want it (like our thighs), and disappears from places where it could benefit our appearance (like our faces).

But there is hope! Start exercising if you aren't already, sure, but there is even more you can do to get your curves in the right places again. In this chapter, let's check in with your body. We'll talk about fat and where it's going, and flab and why it's hanging, and I'll even give you some sound advice on what you can do about aging body skin, drooping breasts, and even some options for those of you who wish your breasts or your butt was just a little bit bigger and fuller than it is right now.

FAT ACCUMULATION

Just about everybody has a beef with the fat that has accumulated in some unwanted spot. Women often tell me they want to get rid of the fat from their abdomens, buttocks, or thighs, while men are more interested in blasting their beer gut or trimming those love handles. Our bodies all deposit fat in their own individual ways, largely due to genetic propensity, and even in very fit people, there can be extra fat. *Always try diet and exercise first*, but in cases where unwanted fat pockets just don't seem to respond to diet and exercise, there are some other good options.

CoolSculpting

Fat-reduction therapies have come a long way in the past several years. Just seven years ago, there was no safe, proven way to reduce fat without surgery. Today, there are over a dozen treatments that claim to reduce fat, and several that are scientifically proven to work. Let's take a look.

As of this writing, CoolSculpting is probably the gold standard for noninvasive fat reduction. This treatment is based on the fact that the skin is more resilient to injury than the fat below it. Knowing this, the CoolSculpting device was created to freeze the skin and the fat underneath it, causing irreversible damage to the fat cells but leaving the skin unharmed. Studies show that one treatment (lasting typically an hour) reduces the thickness of fat by approximately 25 percent. The treatment is virtually painless, but results can take a month or two to show up.

CoolSculpting is a great option for people who want to modestly reduce the fat of their abdomen, hips, waist, or thighs and don't want to undergo surgery. It definitely works and is an ❄️ AGE FIX FAVORITE . My only reservations for this treatment are that the results aren't nearly as dramatic as those achieved with liposuction, and it's quite expensive. Most CoolSculpting centers charge at least $700 per area. This can add up to many thousands of dollars if you want multiple areas treated. However, the treatment is very easily tolerated and doesn't usually necessitate any downtime or cause posttreatment pain.

Liposonix

Another scientifically proven treatment to noninvasively reduce fat is Liposonix. Liposonix uses ultrasound energy, the same ultrasound that is used to look inside a pregnant woman's tummy at a baby inside, but turns that ultrasound energy way up to blast away fat cells. The company advertises its treatment with the promise that you need only one hour-long treatment to lose one inch or one dress size. Scientific studies show that the treatment does, in fact, destroy some of the fat cells in the deeper fat. As with CoolSculpting, the body naturally clears the fat from your body and results can take a month or two to be noticeable. Although I recommend CoolSculpting as the gold standard of noninvasive fat reduction, Liposonix is another valid option with pretty comparable results. According to RealSelf.com, the average cost of Liposonix is $2,450.

UltraShape

UltraShape, like Liposonix, uses ultrasound energy to permanently reduce fat. It's been effectively used for many years outside the United States and was FDA-cleared in 2014 for noninvasive fat reduction. The treatment is virtually painless, and studies show it takes an average of four centimeters off the circumference of the abdomen. Not bad! One big difference between Ultrashape and CoolSculpting or Liposonix is that it takes three treatments, spaced every two weeks, for optimal results. The other treatments just take one, so for this reason I generally recommend CoolSculpting and Liposonix over UltraShape. According to RealSelf.com, the average cost of UltraShape is $2,125.

Radiofrequency Devices

Another method for nonsurgically reducing fat involves radiofrequency devices. These reduce fat by heating it with radiofrequency waves. You may remember that I already told you how radiofrequency waves can heat up and tighten skin. When these waves are turned way up, they can bypass the skin to heat and disrupt the fatty layer underneath.

I initially noticed the ability of radiofrequency to melt fat as an inadvertent consequence of skin-tightening radiofrequency treatments back in 2004. I saw a handful of patients who underwent skin-tightening radiofrequency treatments to their faces by other doctors but were left with faces that looked gaunt or hollow, and even had dents. I treated them by injecting fat into their faces to replump them. I wrote this up in a scientific article for *Plastic and Reconstructive Surgery* in 2007 and reported it on my blog. The company behind the radiofrequency device then had their attorney send me a threatening letter as a result. Now, several years later, the radiofrequency companies have begun to utilize what I helped discover, and are now marketing their devices as fat reducers!

Although these radiofrequency devices can, indeed, reduce fat, in general their results aren't as proven or reliable as CoolSculpting or Liposonix. However, unlike CoolSculpting and Liposonix, these radiofrequency treatments can do more than just reduce fat. They also modestly tighten the skin and smooth cellulite. I describe these devices as "souped-up" cellulite machines to my patients. They may not be as consistently effective in reducing fat as the treatments above, but they have the added benefits of skin smoothing and tightening that CoolSculpting, Liposonix, and UltraShape lack. Unfortunately, these devices necessitate multiple treatments, sometimes as many as eight treatments spaced one week apart, for best results. Some examples of radiofrequency devices that can smooth cellulite, tighten skin, and reduce fat are the **Body FX** (an 🌸 AGE FIX FAVORITE), **VelaShape III**, **truSculpt**, and **Venus Freeze**. If you're interested in a combination of skin tightening, cellulite smoothing, and modest fat reduction, then one of these treatments may be good for you. Costs vary, depending on the number of treatments you have and the device used, but a series of treatments for any of these devices typically starts at $1,000 and up.

Vanquish is the name of a radiofrequency-based fat-reducing device that is completely different from the ones I described above. Unlike the other radiofrequency-based fat reducers, Vanquish doesn't necessitate any contact with the skin. It's used primarily to reduce inches from the midsection, with one study revealing an average loss of two inches after a series of four 30-minute treatments. For the most part, Vanquish treatments are painless, although you may feel some heating of the treated areas. If you are interested in noninvasive reduction of fat from your abdomen and hips, then I'd put CoolSculpting or Vanquish at the top of your list. According to RealSelf.com, the average cost for a set of Vanquish treatments is $2,400.

Low-Light Lasers

The **Zerona** device was the first FDA-cleared, noninvasive fat-removing device. I was one of the first to introduce this game-changing machine on TV back in 2009. The Zerona is a strange-looking contraption that resembles Dr. Octopus from the Spider-Man comic books. It utilizes four low-light lasers, which, after six treatments over two weeks, are believed to cause your fat cells to open up and release their contents. Low-light lasers aren't like the lasers we use to burn facial skin or that we use in surgery. They don't create any heat, which is why they are also called cold lasers. They are better compared to the lasers in laser pointers.

Studies show that patients lose an average of three to four inches when measuring four body parts: each thigh, waist, and hips. We used the device in my office for about a year and found variable results. Some patients lost virtually nothing, whereas others lost as much as eight inches. One big drawback was the lack of control we had over where the inches would come off. The patient might have huge thighs she wanted reduced, but the four inches could instead come off her hips. The Zerona is also now cleared by the FDA for reducing arm circumference as well. In order to encourage and accommodate the body to naturally dispose of the fatty content of these cells, you're encouraged to take niacin supplements, drink plenty of water, and exercise to complement the treatments.

Other devices that use low-light (or cold) lasers are the **i-Lipo** and the **Strawberry Laser Lipo**. In general, low-light laser treatments aren't my top choices for noninvasive fat reduction. Although I believe they work, the results are too variable for me to strongly recommend them.

Mesotherapy

Mesotherapy is a controversial technique that involves injecting a substance under the skin that is caustic to fat. Another name for this treatment is injection lipolysis. This treatment originated in Europe and has since been practiced throughout the world. Although it sounds like a good idea, there are some major concerns regarding the safety and effectiveness of mesotherapy.

One major problem is that there is no standardization about what and how much of it should be injected under the skin to destroy the underlying fat. Basically, any doctor can concoct his or her own witches' brew of caustic substances that may result in the fat dying off. In the mid-2000s, this lack of regulation led many doctors (mostly non–plastic surgeons who wanted to get a big name in the marketplace) to advertise their own mesotherapy treatments. Countless stories of frightening complications ensued, such as infections, tissue death, and disfigurement. Since then, several countries, such as Brazil, have banned mesotherapy.

This hasn't closed the door on a possible safe option in mesotherapy, however. **Kybella** is a new injectable treatment that was FDA-approved in April 2015 for reducing the fat under the chin. It's currently the only effective option (short of liposuction) to thin a double chin. It involves several tiny injections of a substance that is caustic to the fat, irreversibly damaging it and causing the area to gradually thin over several months. The results appear to be permanent! Up to six treatments are necessary, and as of this writing, the cost is still to be determined. Keep in mind that although it appears to be very effective in reducing a double chin, it doesn't tighten the skin. It only removes the fat. Still, I'm very excited about this one.

By the time you read this, I expect everywhere through the United States plastic surgeons and dermatologists will be injecting Kybella. Say hello to my little friend and good-bye to your double chin!

Body Wraps

Short of diet and exercise, there really aren't any at-home ways to permanently reduce fat. Laser manufacturers have made at-home devices for acne, skin rejuvenation, and hair removal, but unfortunately they have yet to introduce anything for the home user that effectively spot-reduces fat. The best thing I've seen that does work, however, is body wraps.

If you want to reduce inches virtually in an instant, such as right before an important function, like a class reunion, a hot date, or a red carpet event, or any time you really want to look a little bit slimmer than you really are, I recommend a body wrap. **Suddenly Slender** is one relatively popular company with franchises across the country. Although these wraps are more commonly performed in spas, they can also be performed at home. They work by draining away excess water weight and can temporarily take off inches within a matter of hours. Many of the manufacturers also claim that their wraps remove the dreaded but vague "toxins." I suppose you sweat a lot during these treatments, and some toxins are always released in sweat. Keep in mind that the results of body wraps aren't permanent, but they can be pretty dramatic.

An easy body wrap for the abdomen and hips that you can do at home is the **Adonia Tummy Tone**. This is a cream composed of organic essential oils and capsaicin that can create rapid (but temporary) inch loss. You generously apply the cream to your abdomen, then have someone wrap your abdomen with plastic wrap (like Saran Wrap) tightly four times around your tummy, like a tight girdle. Lie down on your bed or couch and cover the area with a warm blanket. Read a book, take a nap, or watch some TV. An hour later, unwrap your abdomen and it should be one to two inches smaller. Like other body wraps, this treatment probably works by reducing the excess water in your tissues, causing you to be temporarily smaller for a few hours. Not bad for an hour of lying down and doing nothing!

Insider Tip

Not all fat can be removed with the treatments I have described in this chapter. In general, our bodies put fat in two compartments: subcutaneous and intra-abdominal. Subcutaneous fat is fat that is below the skin and above the muscle. This is fat that you can pinch between your fingers. Intra-abdominal fat lives underneath the muscle layer inside our bellies and surrounds many of our internal organs, such as the intestines. This is the fat that creates a potbelly and is considered dangerous to our health.

So how do you know if your fat is subcutaneous or intra-abdominal? If you can pinch the fat between your fingers, it's subcutaneous. Subcutaneous fat can be reduced by liposuction and the other noninvasive treatments I described in this chapter. If, however, your tummy protrudes and is firm when you poke at it, then you likely have intra-abdominal fat. A propensity for intra-abdominal fat can be passed along from parent to child. I've seen many patients who've unfortunately inherited their potbellies from their moms or dads. Sorry, but the only way to reduce this type of fat is good old-fashioned diet and exercise.

Liposuction

Yes, it's surgery, and yes, it's an apparently easy way to get the fat off. It's not for everyone, but since its introduction to the world of plastic surgery in the 1980s, liposuction is still considered the gold standard for permanent fat reduction. It's certainly not the only scientifically proven way to reduce fat, as we've seen. However, many of my patients are very interested in liposuction, so let's talk about it first, just in case you really want to know.

There are three types of liposuction: tumescent, ultrasonic, and laser:

1. **Tumescent liposuction** is the technique that most plastic surgeons use when they perform liposuction. This procedure involves two steps. First, the surgeon makes a small incision in the skin and injects anesthetic fluid to decrease postoperative pain and limit bleeding. Next, the plastic surgeon uses a long, hollow rod (called a cannula) hooked up to a suction device to mechanically disrupt the deep fat and literally suck it out. The fat that is removed is gone. Permanently. The patient is placed into a spandex garment to decrease swelling and bleeding, which he or she wears for the next three to four weeks. This is typically a very efficient way to permanently remove fat cells from the body.

2. **Ultrasonic liposuction** was developed in the late 1990s and currently goes by brand names such as **Vaser** and **Lysonix**. The first step (infusion of anesthetic) is the same, and the last step (sucking out the fat) is the same as in the tumescent technique, but there is a middle step. In the middle step, the surgeon inserts an ultrasonic cannula, which looks similar to the liposuction cannula except that the end emits ultrasonic energy. This allows the plastic surgeon to melt fat and connective tissue fibers and theoretically remove fat more efficiently. It can help a surgeon more effectively remove fat from areas where it is dense and fibrous (like a man's breast or in a person with a lot of scar tissue), but at added expense and the rare risk of burns. I rarely use ultrasonic liposuction anymore, since its benefits for most people overall are pretty minimal.

3. **Laser liposuction** was developed most recently, over the past several years, and goes by the brand names **Smart Lipo**, **Slim Lipo**, **LipoLite**, and others. In this surgery, the first and last steps (infusion of anesthetic and sucking out the fat) are the same as in tumescent liposuction, but, like ultrasonic liposuction, there is a middle step. In laser liposuction the plastic surgeon takes a thin laser fiber and passes it under the skin numerous times, in order to heat up the skin overlying the fat. Theoretically, the heat causes the skin to tighten. The big question is: How much does the skin actually tighten? It depends on whom you ask. Doctors who own the laser liposuction devices often claim that the skin tightening can be dramatic. Doctors who don't own the devices often claim there is no tightening at all. I suspect that the truth is likely somewhere in between but probably leaning more toward the little-to-no-tightening side. My recommendation is that if you are considering paying extra for laser liposuction, choose a small area where even a modicum of skin tightening will be noticeable and worth the additional expense. This could include the skin under your chin and your arms. The Smart Lipo device arguably has the most safety mechanisms built in, so the risk of burns is lower with this device than with the others. So if you choose to have laser liposuction, I recommend that you find a board-certified plastic surgeon who uses Smart Lipo.

So should you have liposuction? Which type of liposuction is best for you? If you have small, stubborn areas of fat that are resistant to diet and exercise, and the cost and invasiveness of liposuction aren't deterrents, then you may be a good candidate for the procedure. Ninety percent or more of people who are good candidates for liposuction do just fine with the tumescent technique, saving time and money in the process. If you've had liposuction before and need a second revision procedure, then ultrasonic liposuction may be right for you. If you just want to reduce fat in a small area (such as under the chin or the upper arms) and have a little loose skin, then it may be wise to look into laser liposuction, specifically Smart Lipo.

The cost of liposuction varies, typically starting at about $1,000 for a small area to $10,000-plus for extensive liposuction. Adding ultrasonic or laser to the procedure also adds costs, which could run in the thousands of dollars.

Keep in mind that liposuction isn't a weight-loss procedure and is not a valid substitute for diet and exercise. The maximum amount of fat that the FDA recommends to be removed in one outpatient setting is about five liters, or eleven pounds of fat. Anything more than this can be dangerous, with the potential need for blood transfusions.

And did I mention trying diet and exercise first?

Caution!

Liposuction should not be performed on thin people. Almost every day I have a person ask me to liposuction an area with very little fat in the first place. Contrary to popular belief, liposuction does not cause problem areas to look smoother. It can actually do the exact opposite of this, especially in people without much fat to remove. The scar tissue that results from liposuction can leave unnatural-looking dents in people who don't have enough fat left behind to camouflage it. You can definitely be too skinny for liposuction!

We've gone over many options to permanently reduce fat. Here is a summary of what I recommend, depending on what you are hoping to achieve:

* Modest fat reduction of abdomen, love handles, hips, and waist: **CoolSculpting** or **Vanquish**

* Modest fat reduction of thighs: **CoolSculpting** or **UltraShape**

* Modest fat reduction with skin tightening and cellulite reduction of the buttocks and/or thighs: **Body FX**, **VelaShape III**, **truSculpt**, or **Venus Freeze**

* Dramatic fat reduction for most problem areas: **tumescent liposuction** (in general, you can't go wrong with this)

* Dramatic fat reduction with skin tightening under the chin: **laser liposuction** (ideally with Smart Lipo)

CELLULITE

Cellulite is that bumpy fat just under the skin, and it is the bane of many an existence come swimsuit season. Cellulite forms because fat under the skin is separated by fibrous bands, called septae, into compartments. If the fat expands and the septae remain tight and stiff, then the fat shows up in the dimples we know as cellulite. Unlike pockets of fat that appear where you don't want them to, cellulite tends to spread out over the backs of thighs, on the buttocks, on the tummy, or even around the upper arms. It doesn't stick out as much as it just looks like, well…cottage cheese.

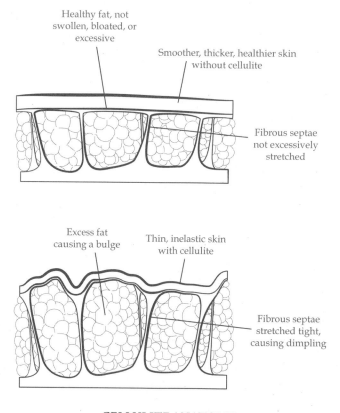

Healthy fat, not swollen, bloated, or excessive

Smoother, thicker, healthier skin without cellulite

Fibrous septae not excessively stretched

Excess fat causing a bulge

Thin, inelastic skin with cellulite

Fibrous septae stretched tight, causing dimpling

CELLULITE ANATOMY

Companies have been coming up with anticellulite treatments for years, and most of them don't work very well. However, there are a few that do work. But first let's talk about the surgical option. You may not go for this, but I want you to know it exists.

Cellulaze

Cellulaze is the first and only FDA-approved surgical treatment for cellulite reduction. The procedure entails use of a small laser fiber that is tunneled underneath the skin. The laser fires its beams sideways, causing the fibrous septae that cause cellulite to be disturbed. By breaking apart the fibers that make the fat form into dimples, you get a smoother surface. The fat is still there, but it looks more like cream than cottage cheese, which is a much more preferable option for many people. The results appear to be long lasting, and while there is no permanent cure for cellulite, so far this seems to be the closest thing we have to it. This is surgery, however, and it can be a costly procedure. According to RealSelf.com, the average cost of Cellulaze is $5,825.

Heating Technology

If you would rather have a professional tackle your cellulite but you don't want surgery, you have a few good options, and all of them are based on the same principle: combining a warming up of the underlying fat and a deep-tissue massage to stretch the septae. Where the treatments differ most is in how the fat is heated:

* **SmoothShapes** heats the fat with lasers.

* **Dermosonic** heats the fat with ultrasound.

* **VelaShape**, **Venus Freeze**, **truSculpt**, and **Body FX** heat the fat with radiofrequency.

* **Endermologie** doesn't heat the fat at all. Instead, it relies on deep massage using a specialized body suit.

The good thing about these in-office treatments is that they don't hurt, have no downtime, and actually are effective. The bad thing is that results are temporary and necessitate multiple treatments spaced one to two weeks apart. This can get costly.

Still, I like some of them. The newest treatments, as I mentioned earlier, are even creating skin tightening and some modest inch loss as well.

Wellbox

This is another cellulite treatment device, but this one you can use at home. It's similar to Endermologie in the way it works. This involves a deep-tissue massage on your thighs and buttocks, causing them to smooth within a few treatments. There are no permanent cures for cellulite, but this can be a nice substitute for thousands of dollars of in-office cellulite treatments. The device costs about $1,200 to $1,500, depending on where you get it.

Adonia LegTone Serum

You've probably seen cellulite creams at the drugstore and wondered whether they worked. Frankly, many of them don't do much of anything, but there are a few that I think offer some nice results, even if they are less dramatic than some of the options I've talked about already. One of my ✺ AGE FIX FAVORITES is Adonia LegTone Serum. It smooths cellulite with visible results in just nine minutes. It's composed of plant-derived stem cells and twenty-three organic essential oils. You need to apply it twice a day for the first two months, after which your cellulite should be significantly improved. After this, apply only once a day. The company's studies show a 47 percent reduction in cellulite after just two applications, and a 72 percent reduction in cellulite after six weeks of use. My employees pooh-poohed this cream, but after using it they were surprised at how well it worked! You can purchase a sixty-day supply online for about $80.

DIY Cellulite Treatment

Caffeine can reduce the swelling that accentuates cellulite, so for those of you who like to try DIY treatments, try a scrub made out of coffee grounds. Massage a half cup of brewed (and still wet) coffee grounds onto your skin. Apply plastic wrap over this area, allowing it to hold some of the grounds against your skin for ten minutes. It should have an immediate and temporary but relatively long-lasting (six to ten hours) result.

THE SKIN ON YOUR BODY

We all tend to focus on the quality, tightness, color, smoothness, and softness of the face, but we have a whole lot of other skin that can get rough, discolored, droopy, and wrinkled, which can accentuate or even change body shape in a way we may not like. As we age, skin takes a beating, especially the skin exposed to the sun and elements, as well as the skin that gets stretched out through childbirth or weight gain, or droops after childbirth or with massive weight loss. Body skin can get rough patches and age spots and even calluses and a rough, wrinkly texture, and that can make anybody look older. Once they reach their sixties, many people who have aggressively fought aging all their lives may decide to throw in the towel when it comes to fighting drooping and aging on areas other than the face, especially the breasts, tummy, and hands.

However, there are ways to rejuvenate the skin on the body. Plastic surgeons lift these areas with breast lifts, tummy tucks, and lasers to the hands, but this is more difficult with loose skin and sun damage on the legs, back, arms, buttocks, and (ahem) genitals. I've joked with my patients that if I could invent a full-body laser that tightened up the skin head to toe, then I would make a fortune. It would be crafted like a CT scanner; a person's entire body would go through the device, which would tighten up the skin as it went. I can see just how it would work! Alas, there is no such thing, and no laser company is interested in developing the device and giving me credit. Fortunately, we do have some other options for improving the skin on your body. First, let's talk about skin quality, color, and softness.

KojiLac-CHQ Pads

This product is my 🌸 AGE FIX FAVORITE for improving the smoothness of the skin of our bodies, and it also helps eliminate dark spots. These are sold only in the offices of certain doctors, but if you can find a physician (probably a plastic surgeon or dermatologist) who carries them, I recommend giving them a try. These pads are specifically made for body rather than face skin. They look like larger versions of those acne pads you buy in jars, but these are infused with a potent combination of kojic acid and hydroquinone, both skin lighteners, as well as the antioxidants vitamin C and green tea, and lactic acid, which is an alpha-hydroxy acid. These ingredients reduce age spots, exfoliate the skin, and fight off free-radical damage so the skin on your body looks younger. Not bad for an over-the-counter product!

DIY Body-Beautifying Baths

An all-natural method for improving the skin quality of the whole body is a **green tea bath**. Although this won't actually change your shape, it can make your skin look younger. Steep five green tea bags in your bathwater, then soak for fifteen to twenty minutes. The antioxidants in the tea will rejuvenate your skin, and the caffeine can provide a nice temporary tightening effect as well. If you throw in a few lemon slices, you get the added benefit of an antioxidant boost from vitamin C.

Another option is the **milk bath**. Add one or two cups of powdered milk to your warm bathwater. The lactic acid in the milk will provide for very gentle chemical exfoliation. If your skin is oily, use nonfat powdered milk. If your skin is dry, try powdered whole milk. For even greater benefit, add those green tea bags to the water, too.

Exfoliating your face can help to reveal younger skin, and you can get the same effect all over your body if you have the right tool. This reminds me of the Korean sandpaperlike washcloths that my mom put in our showers and bathtubs when I was growing up. Instead of loofah sponges and soft washcloths, we used the equivalent of a sandblaster on our skin. I remember that these washcloths would leave my skin feeling like one big, bloody abrasion. It felt like I'd just fallen off a motorcycle at sixty miles an hour on a gravel road while naked. Although the washcloths of my childhood were a bit too aggressive, I do think the Koreans were on to something. Mechanical exfoliation is probably the easiest way to soften and smooth the skin of our bodies. I just don't recommend something that would leave a scar!

Instead of going to a Korean drugstore to look for washcloths, I suggest using a kitchen sponge in the shower. Get the kind with a spongy side and the darker, rough side for scrubbing counters and sinks. Use the rough side to exfoliate your body, being especially aggressive with the bottoms of your feet. The spongy side can be used on more delicate areas, like the face and genitals.

LOOSE TUMMY SKIN

Improving skin quality is great, but sometimes you need a more powerful effect than you can get through exfoliation and moisturizing. When skin droops, it is a sure sign of aging (or at least of some big experience, like childbirth or a huge weight loss), and of all the places that droop, tummy droop seems to distress people the most. But can you do anything about it?

The skin of the tummy (and the underlying muscles and tissues surrounding the muscles) gets stretched out during pregnancy or with excessive weight gain, and in most people, it never completely shrinks back into place after birth or weight loss. In mild cases, it can cause an accordionlike look to the skin when bending over, due to the multiple folds the loose skin produces. In the most severe cases the skin can hang over the pubic area, otherwise known as the dreaded pannus or panniculus. This can happen after pregnancy as well as after massive weight loss.

I can't tell you how many women have asked me for a nonsurgical solution to loose tummy skin. Lasers and other devices like radiofrequency treatments have been used to tighten this skin, all with disappointing results. Theoretically, these devices would tighten body skin in the same way they tighten the skin of the face, but the problem is that the only ones that seem to have even moderately noticeable results are both painful and expensive. The ones that don't have any pain associated with them have minimal or no results, in my experience. As of this writing, I'm still waiting for the body-tightening laser that actually is worth the money. I hate to tell you this, but I want you to know the truth: At this time, the only effective solution for loose tummy skin is an actual tummy tuck.

Tummy Tuck

A tummy tuck may sound awesome—a simple surgery to get rid of your droopy stomach? Before you sign up, though, there are some things you should know. The tummy tuck is an invasive surgery that takes anywhere from two to four hours to perform and has a two- to three-week recovery period. This surgery, usually performed under general anesthesia, allows the surgeon to perform two main tasks: removing the excess skin and fat from the tummy and tightening the underlying muscle layer.

Here's how it works: The plastic surgeon removes all the skin from between the pubic area and the belly button by making a hip-to-hip incision (and resulting scar), lifting the skin and fat off the underlying muscle layer, cutting off the excess skin and fat (typically everything between the belly button and the pubic area), and pulling the skin above the belly button down to the pubic region. The belly button is retained but is now surrounded by skin that used to be much higher on the tummy. The muscle tightening involves using permanent or semipermanent sutures to stitch the stretched-out muscles back together, kind of like an internal corset. This part of the surgery causes the most discomfort. Like I said, it's pretty invasive.

Caution!

If you hear about some yahoo doctor advertising his or her own version of a tummy tuck that is supposedly better than the tummy tucks of other plastic surgeons, don't believe the hype. It's just not true. If it were, then I (and thousands of my reputable colleagues) would do it, too.

The tummy tuck leaves a hip-to-hip scar and a round scar around the belly button that are both permanent. These scars never go away, even when you reach your ninety-fifth birthday. A good plastic surgeon will do his or her best to position the lower scar so it is hidden underneath clothing, like shorts or even a two-piece bathing suit. I call my tummy tuck a Hidden Scar Tummy Tuck for this very reason. However, these scars will always be visible to you, and could be to anyone else who sees you without clothing.

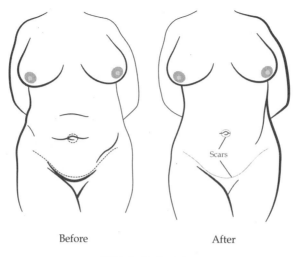

Before   After

TUMMY TUCK

Interestingly, however, although tummy tucks are one of the more invasive cosmetic surgeries that plastic surgeons perform, they also have one of the highest satisfaction rates. For some patients, getting rid of the excess, hanging skin of the tummy is well worth the expense and discomfort of the surgery. Until we develop my incredible skin-shrinking laser, it's either tummy tuck or nothing. (Attention, laser companies: Call me!)

Celeb Spot

One celebrity who admitted that she had a tummy tuck and loved the results was Kate Gosselin (of *Kate Plus 8*). Although bikini photos of her in *Us Weekly* revealed a barely visible scar, she still looked amazing.

AGING, SHRINKING, OR DEFLATED BREASTS

Unfortunately, aging, and especially aging combined with a history of childbirth, does a number on a woman's breasts. Skin loses elasticity with age, and the thick, firm breast tissue of youth gets replaced by soft, shapeless fat, especially after having children and going through menopause. Breast-feeding can cause the breasts to undergo massive fluctuations in size, which stretches out the skin. Gravity works every second of every minute of every day to pull breasts downward. That's why, when you're young and your breasts are perky, it's important to wear a supportive bra. This helps prevent gravity from exerting its influence on your breasts all day long.

As you age, however, bras can help but only so much, and when you take them off, all bets are off. Aging breasts can definitely contribute to looking and feeling older, especially if your breasts look nothing like they used to. Aging changes all body parts to some extent, but most of my patients who come in for breast-related issues are women over thirty (and some in their seventies) who just want to reclaim some of what their breasts used to look like. They aren't twenty-two-year-olds who want double Ds. They just want to feel like themselves again.

There are several key issues with aging and breasts. Let's start with drooping.

Droopy Breasts

If your breasts seem to be sinking closer and closer to your navel with every passing year, you have a very common condition. Gravity and weakening skin often lead to drooping. In fact, just about every woman over the age of fifty with a C cup or higher has droopy breasts. This is just part of nature and time. If your breasts are droopy, what can you do about it? Here are some options.

CAFFEINE

You can attain a more modest lift at home simply by using a skin-tightening cream containing caffeine. There are many commercially available creams that contain caffeine and are used as firming creams for the thighs and buttocks, but that also work on the breasts. One popular cream, **Fat Girl Slim**, can be purchased at Sephora. If you can get over the irreverent name, you might want to try it. I've seen caffeine products result in improvement that you should be able to see and feel. Keep in mind, though, that the tightening is temporary. The only way to get a permanent lift is with surgery (and scars). Bummer, right?

Beauty Secret

Although cosmetics can't make your breasts perkier or larger, they can enhance the overall effect. Try this cosmetic fix:

1. First, get your breasts at the level you want them—boost them up by putting on a cleavage-enhancing bra.

2. Using a bronzer product or a foundation a few shades darker than your skin, brush or blend a subtle arc over the top of your breasts and along the inner cleavage, from cleavage to bra strap, giving the illusion of more fullness.

3. Using highlighter, brush above and below the bronzer and in the space between your breasts, so it looks like a shadow. Blend everything gently so it doesn't look fake.

4. Cover with a layer of shimmery powder to dazzle the eye and further blur the makeup lines.

5. Go out on the town—your cleavage looks awesome!

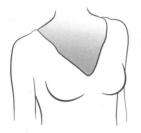

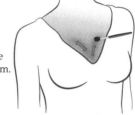

Step 1. Wear a cleavage-enhancing bra.

Step 2. Brush bronzer over the tops of your breasts and along the inner cleavage to outline them.

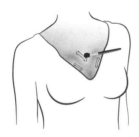

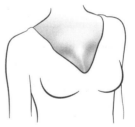

Step 3. Brush highlighter above and below the bronzer, and in the space between your breasts. Blend it gently.

Step 4. Cover with a layer of shimmery powder.

ENHANCE BREASTS WITH MAKEUP

BREAST LIFT

Of course there is also a surgical option, and it has proven quite popular in Hollywood. Nobody *needs* a breast lift, also called a mastopexy. You can always boost the "girls" with a supportive bra as you get older and leave it at that. However, if your drooping breasts really bother you, if they have moved significantly south on your chest and you are constantly feeling the urge to pull them up and you really do think surgery would help, you should know what you are getting into first. The mastopexy is typically a two- to three-hour operation. During it, the surgeon removes the excess skin of the droopy breasts, and the nipples and remaining breast tissue are repositioned up the chest where they once were. This might sound fairly straightforward, and the surgery definitely works well, but there is one catch. One big catch. You get major scars from this surgery.

The scars from a breast lift vary in length depending on just how droopy you are. If your droopiness is fairly minimal, sometimes the lift can be done with a scar that just extends circumferentially around your areola (the colored circle around your nipple). With moderate droopiness, a lollipop scar can be used, where the scar extends circumferentially around your areola but also extends vertically downward to the crease under your breasts. Severe droopiness often necessitates an "anchor" scar, which is a lollipop scar plus a horizontal scar extending along the crease under your breasts. These scars can be quite extensive, and they are also permanent. They will never go away. When you are eighty-five years old, the scars from your breast lift you got in your forties will still be there, albeit likely quite faded.

Many women ask me if breast implants can lift their breasts. Unfortunately, implants do not have magical hovering properties. In fact, they do the exact opposite. Breast implants make your breasts heavier, causing gravity to pull them downward even more, which results in your breasts drooping even more quickly.

In other words, breast implants make your breasts larger but don't lift them. Breast lifts will lift your breasts but won't make them bigger. Deciding to have breast surgery means deciding what your priority is.

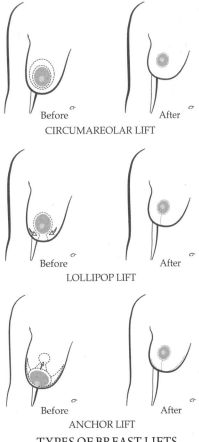

Before — After
CIRCUMAREOLAR LIFT

Before — After
LOLLIPOP LIFT

Before — After
ANCHOR LIFT
TYPES OF BREAST LIFTS

BREAST AUGMENTATION

If your problem isn't so much droopiness as it is flatness—the deflated breasts that so often come with age, where breasts lose volume, fullness, and roundness, you may be one of the many women interested in breast augmentation. Or maybe you have always had small breasts and always wished for more, and now that you are more established in your career, you can finally afford the breast augmentation surgery you always wanted. Small breasts are, of course, perfectly lovely and many people prefer them. They stay perky longer and don't droop as easily, they don't get in the way when you exercise (or sleep on your stomach), and many people like the way they look. For some people, however, small breasts don't feel right or balanced for their bodies, and they truly believe they will feel better with an adjustment.

Before you consider surgery, you should know that short of gaining weight and hoping it goes topside, there is one nonsurgical breast augmentation option that works fairly well.

Brava: **Brava** is the only scientifically proven, FDA-cleared method of breast enhancement without surgery. Studies show it can add 150 cc of size to each breast, which is about one-half to one-third the size of an average breast implant. It's a modest gain and not as dramatic as surgery, but it is measurable.

Brava works by the process of tissue expansion. The device has two large suction cups that attach to the breasts and apply constant suction to the breasts, causing them to be stretched larger. Studies show they can actually cause new breast tissue to be created. However, you must wear the device at least ten hours each night. Studies show that after ten to fourteen weeks you can get an average of a one-cup increase in breast size. It's tedious and difficult to stick with the program, though. If you miss just one night, then you lose a significant portion of the results. The cost of Brava is about $1,200.

Some doctors are combining this treatment with fat injections for a much greater increase in breast size. However, the fat injections entail actual surgery, and there is some controversy regarding whether the fat injections may alter mammograms. For this reason, it's not something I recommend unless breast implants just aren't an option.

This may sound like too much work and expense to you, and I agree. Brava can work, but this is one of the few cases where surgery really does give results far and away better than nonsurgical treatments. But what about creams or natural methods of breast enhancement? There really isn't an effective way to make your breasts bigger using natural, at-home ingredients. And the many creams sold online that claim to make the breasts bigger don't seem to work, either. They simply aren't worth the money.

For some people, surgery is.

BREAST IMPLANTS

Surgery certainly isn't everyone's choice, nor should it be. However, breast augmentation surgery is the most popular plastic surgery on the planet. For women who get a modest augmentation, it is straightforward and often looks very natural. It comprises about one-third of my plastic surgery practice, and I perform over 150 breast augmentation surgeries every year. According to the American Society for Aesthetic Plastic Surgery (ASAPS), each year more than 300,000 women undergo breast augmentation surgery. That reveals a lot of discontent about breasts, and a lot of effort and money to increase their size. Many celebrities have even come forward and admitted having breast implants, including Kelly Rowland of Destiny's Child, Denise Richards, and Jane Seymour.

Maybe you are one of the many women interested in this procedure. I'm certainly not going to try to convince you that you should get this surgery, or that you shouldn't. Breast size and fullness are very personal matters. However, I know from my practice that many women have considered this, especially as they age and their breasts change. If this is you, then I want to give you the information you need so you know exactly what you are considering. So let's talk, surgeon to reader, about breast augmentation.

Size Matters: First of all, you should know what size you want to be. Contrary to popular belief, almost no one asks for gigantic breasts. Most women want to look natural, with the most common request going from an A cup to a C cup in size. That being said, women start and end at all sizes. However, implants don't come in A, B, C, and D cup sizes like bras. Instead, they are measured in milliliters.

The easiest way to determine what size is right for you is to use a tester, or **sizer implants**. Most plastic surgery offices have implants of all different sizes that you can put into a bra to determine how they will look on you. I recommend that you put a plain T-shirt over the bra to really get a good idea of how you will look afterward.

The other way women are deciding implant sizes is with **computerized 3-D imaging**. This is a specialized device that takes a 3-D picture of your chest and allows you to see an estimation of how your chest will look with various-sized implants. Their accuracy in predicting your outcome is usually pretty good. The most popular 3-D imaging devices are the **Vectra**, the **Axis 3D**, and the **Crisalix**.

When choosing the appropriate size of breast implant for you, keep in mind that the bigger the implant, the quicker it will droop. I've seen many, many women with really large breast implants put in by other doctors that have resulted in premature drooping of the breasts. Plastic surgeons sometimes call this bottoming out. So choose your size wisely, and don't go bigger than you need to!

Just Your Type: The next thing to consider is what type of implant to use. This is the most common question I get. Back in the 1980s and early 1990s, most women underwent breast augmentation with **liquid silicone implants**. These implants had two major problems. The outer shell was really weak, causing them to break quite often, and the silicone inside the implants was a liquid, which would ooze out of any break in the implant shell. When this occurred it created a mess, sometimes with excess scar tissue and inflammation.

Because of this, many women were concerned that their implants were causing various diseases, such as lupus, arthritis, and even breast cancer. In response to this fear, in 1992 the FDA banned the use of silicone breast implants, allowing them only in strictly controlled studies. However, these studies showed no connection between silicone breast implants and any disease, prompting the FDA to lift the ban on silicone implants in November 2006.

Today, the implants are much improved. The outer shells are much stronger, and very resistant to breakage. The silicone inside the implants is no longer a liquid but a cohesive gel. This is a gel that sticks together and doesn't leak out like the older, liquid silicone implants. For these reasons, we are not as concerned about the new style of breast implants as we were with the older ones. People like this style of implant, because it is soft and feels very natural. However, if the silicone implant does break, it can be very difficult to tell and could require an MRI to diagnose the break. MRIs can be very expensive (costing in the thousands of dollars), and most insurance plans don't cover MRIs to solely look for a broken breast implant.

Another new style of implant is the **gummy bear** breast implant. The scientific term is "form-stable." These implants are also made out of silicone, but they are firmer and made to hold their shape, hence the popular term *gummy bear*. The silicone is more of a solid than a liquid. They aren't as firm as an actual gummy bear, though. Instead, they are made to feel like real breast tissue. The benefit of the gummy bear implants is that the risk of silicone leakage is definitely minimized. They also keep their shape nicely, which can be particularly beneficial for people with little supportive breast tissue to hold the implants up. The downside is that these are the most expensive types of implants. They also don't feel as soft as silicone gel, and if they do break, they can be even harder to diagnose, again possibly necessitating an MRI. Currently, these implants are used most commonly in the United States for breast reconstruction after mastectomy. Some well-respected plastic surgeons use the gummy bear implants for most of their cosmetic patients, too, but my experience is that they feel a bit firmer than most of my patients want.

Caution!

Two caveats to the silicone breast implants (including the gummy bear type) in the United States: You must be at least twenty-two years of age to have them, and the FDA recommends follow-up MRI exams at three years after surgery and every other year thereafter to monitor for breaks and leakage.

A third style of implant is the **saline implant**. These implants are popular because they are less expensive, and because they are filled with salt water, it is easy to tell when the implant breaks and easy to remove and replace them. However, saline implants don't look or feel as natural as the new silicone and gummy bear–style implants. Saline implants tend to have more wrinkles and ripples. Sometimes you really do get what you pay for.

In general, the surgeon, operating room, and anesthesia costs are the same no matter which type of implant you choose. The cost of the actual implants, though, varies. A rule of thumb is that saline implants are the least expensive, cohesive silicone implants are about twice the cost of saline, and gummy bear implants are about three times the cost of saline. According to RealSelf.com, the average cost of breast augmentation surgery is $6,425. Expect to pay a little more for silicone and a little less for saline.

If you aren't thrilled about any of these options, you may want to consider the newest breast implant on the market. I consider it the ideal implant, and that is actually its name: the **Ideal Implant**. This is a saline-filled implant, but it contains inner chambers that are designed to limit the wrinkling and rippling of the implant. It was designed by a plastic surgeon who noticed that while flying in a plane, the ice cubes in his glass of water seemed to limit the sloshing around of the water when the plane hit some turbulence. He discovered that this idea could be applied to breast implants as well.

Some surgeons believe this implant can give the natural feel and look of a silicone implant with the safety of a saline implant. It was approved by the FDA at the end of 2014. Time will tell whether the Ideal Implant will truly live up to its name, but I am very optimistic that it will!

Other Decisions: There are just a few other breast implant decisions you will need to make:

* **Textured shell versus smooth shell:** The outer surface of an implant is made of a type of silicone rubber. The shell can be produced to have either a smooth surface or a rough, textured surface. For most of my patients, I choose smooth surface implants, because they tend to feel softer and more natural. The smooth surface allows the implant to glide around inside the breast pocket. However, textured surfaces are designed to adhere to the implant pocket. This prevents the implant from moving around. I prefer textured implants in patients undergoing breast reconstruction, where the breast tissue has been removed during a mastectomy. The textured surface can help prevent the implant from drooping prematurely, especially since the breast tissue that normally holds an implant in place has been removed.

* **Low versus moderate versus high profile:** Implants come in all different levels of roundness. The low profile is the flattest, widest implant, followed by the moderate, moderate plus, and high. There are now ultrahigh-profile implants, which are really round. You know, in case you are going for that beach ball look.

* **Anatomic versus round:** Implants are also made in two shapes: anatomic (or teardrop) and round. I prefer round implants with smooth surfaces in most first-time breast augmentation patients. The anatomic implants all have textured shells and are made to stick in place. All gummy bear–style implants are textured, anatomic implants. Once again, these can be better for women who are having breast reconstruction after a mastectomy for breast cancer. One main problem with these implants is that if one becomes displaced or turned upside down, you may need another surgery to put it back in the correct position.

The actual breast augmentation takes about one to two hours and is usually performed under a general anesthetic. Recovery time takes between several days and several weeks, depending on the size of the implant used and the technique the surgeon employs. I prefer a technique called **Rapid Recovery Breast Augmentation**, which combines a less traumatic surgical technique with reasonably sized implants. Using a combination of these factors, I find that most of my patients take only a handful of pain pills (if that) and are back to most normal activities within forty-eight to seventy-two hours.

However, not all plastic surgeons employ a rapid recovery technique, so make sure to inquire with your potential surgeon to see whether this may apply to you. Choose your surgeon carefully. See examples of previous work. You'll want to feel comfortable with the person you choose, and you'll want someone with a lot of experience. Know that there are many satisfied women out there. You could be one of them.

Insider Tip

Perhaps you've heard of the **Thai breast slap**. This is a technique developed by the Thai government and Khemmikka Na Songkhla, a breast-slapping specialist. During the Thai breast slap, the breasts are kneaded, like bread dough, and the tissue from the sides is aggressively pushed toward the chest, causing the actual breast tissue to be stretched. A limited study on forty volunteers who underwent the Thai breast slap found that some women's breast sizes increased by four inches. Do I believe it? Not really. And does the Thai breast slap work? I highly doubt it. Theoretically, the breasts could be stretched, but I don't see how this could make the breasts any larger. I can only imagine it would make them droopier. Makes for a weird story, though!

DROOPING OR FLATTENING REAR END

Butts are in. There is no question. The public fascination with the booty began with Jennifer Lopez and has been continued by Kim Kardashian, Beyoncé, Nicki Minaj, and Iggy Azalea. Even Pippa, sister of Princess Kate, has gotten into the act. The dress she wore for the royal wedding in April 2011 reportedly created a spike in butt-enhancement operations, including one Miami-based plastic surgeon coining the term "the Pippa Butt Lift." Now it seems everyone wants to get their butts bigger and more shapely.

However, in many cases, just as with breast augmentation, the patients who come in complaining about their rear view aren't just twenty-year-olds who want to channel J.Lo. They are women in their thirties, forties, and fifties who have noticed that they have lost volume and height back there. Their butts are sagging, drooping, or going curiously flat, and they want to know what they can do to get back some of the volume they used to have.

Of course, you can shape your butt with diet and exercise. Muscle toning alone can do a lot of good back there, but the women who come in asking about rear-end enhancement aren't usually the ones who tend to gain weight in that area with extra cupcakes or super squat sets. They are the ones who have butts that are more naturally flat and that go flatter with age. The first option to try is shapewear, which turns out to be all the lift and volume some people want.

Butt Shapers

Aside from good gluteal exercises or gaining a lot of weight, there really isn't an effective, nonsurgical way to permanently enlarge your butt. However, there are a plethora of girdlelike body shapers that can temporarily give you a ba-donka-donk. They typically come in two types: girdles that have a big hole for each butt cheek to stick out of, or girdles with bike-shorts-like padding to make your buttocks look larger.

For the girdles with holes, **Bubbles Bodywear** makes their "Double O" buttock lifter. These tight undergarments feature a double-O opening, allowing your butt cheeks to protrude out to look round and full.

For the girdles with padding, my friend and famous *Dr. 90210* plastic surgeon Dr. Robert Rey has a shapewear line that features his **Bottom Enhancer**. This elastic undergarment tightens up the lower tummy and thighs but comes with removable foam pads to enlarge the buttocks. It's as good as any other similar ones of its kind, but keep in mind, of course, that once you strip down for your Kim Kardashian–style photo shoot, those pads will be cast aside and you probably won't be able to balance a champagne glass back there. (I really don't know anybody who could. Let's be realistic.)

Butt-Enhancement Surgery

If shapewear simply isn't good enough for you and you really do want to add some permanent volume to your backside, there are, as you may have guessed, some surgical options. They aren't the best surgical options, but they are out there.

The first technique involves the insertion of a **solid silicone butt implant**. It's like a breast implant for your derriere. These large, half-grapefruit-shaped rubbery implants are inserted through an incision in the vertical crease dividing your two buttocks. The surgeon places the implant either above or below the gluteus maximus muscle. It's not a very common surgery and has a relatively high rate of complications. One dreaded complication is infection, because, let's face it, that area is not considered the cleanest part of the body, and do you really want to be hospitalized for a butt infection?

Other complications that can occur include implant displacement (meaning it moves outside of your buttock cheeks into another part of your body, like your lower back), and excess scar tissue around the implant, causing it to feel like a real grapefruit in your booty. A couple of years ago, a woman placed a video on YouTube that showed her buttock implant freely moving around. She could move it side-to-side and even flip it over. The video went viral and she subsequently told her story on the E! network's *Botched*.

One final thing to consider with buttock implants is that it might feel like you are sitting on George Costanza's overstuffed wallet (from the show *Seinfeld*). This is not a pleasant sensation for many people. Perhaps you can tell that I am not a fan of the butt implant.

The other way to enhance the buttocks is with a **Brazilian butt lift**. I'm not sure why it's called a butt lift, because technically it is a buttock augmentation. It doesn't lift the butt at all; it just fills out the butt with your own fat. For this procedure, the plastic surgeon liposuctions fat from one part of your body (typically the tummy, hips, and/or thighs), purifies it, and reinjects it into your behind. Not all of the fat will stay in place, however, as an average of 30–70 percent of it will likely reabsorb and disappear, depending on the technique the doctor uses. This surgery is probably the best way to get a fuller, rounder butt, though, and is performed by many more plastic surgeons than buttock implant surgery.

The drawback to this procedure is the longer surgery time and the fact that your buttock won't necessarily feel firmer after surgery, just bigger. Also, skinny women need not apply. You need a significant amount of fat available to properly plump up the butt. You will also need to avoid sitting on your butt for about a month after the surgery. Yes, this can disrupt your plans to take a long car ride or go to the movie theater, not to mention work at a desk. So do you really need surgical butt augmentation? Probably not. But if you really want it? Now you know the facts.

Your shape is a highly personal matter, and only you can decide what you feel good about, what you can live with, and what you absolutely have to change. Now you know your options. How about a trip to the gym while you consider them? One other benefit of exercise is that it improves both mood and self-esteem. Enough of it might help you not to worry so much about the size of this or the relative volume or height of that. Make exercise a habit, and you just may find that body shape modification isn't as crucial as you thought it was.

9 OTHER YOUTH and BEAUTY ISSUES

Although the majority of my patients come in for common aging issues of the face (like crow's-feet, the 11 sign, or neck droop) or for restoring the curves and shapes of youth (like for concerns about drooping breasts or extra skin), some body issues that many people struggle with are less commonly talked about. If you have them, these issues may be even more likely to impact your self-esteem than wrinkles or cellulite dimples. They aren't dangerous, but they make people very self-conscious, and although they might be present in youth, all of these get worse with age and become more noticeable. The good news is that most of these issues can be resolved without surgery. If you have some issues beyond wrinkles and curves that bother you, then read on—you'll find solutions here.

VEIN ISSUES

We all have veins, and thank goodness for that, but most of us would probably rather not *see* our veins, let alone feel them aching. Yet, problems with visible veins—whether the bulging veins we call varicose veins, or the blue-and-red webs we call spider veins that usually pop up on the legs—are quite common. They tend to worsen with age and pregnancy, as well as with years of standing a lot. If you've been dreading putting on those shorts when the weather warms up because you can't stand to look at those veins, here's what you need to know.

Varicose Veins

Varicose veins are puffy, enlarged veins, typically on the legs (when they occur in the bottom, they are called hemorrhoids—different name, same problem). They can enlarge and even create soreness. They are hardly rare—20 percent of men and 40 percent of women have varicose veins somewhere. Varicose veins are caused by dysfunctional valves in the veins. These valves are supposed to let the blood flow in only one direction, but over time they can weaken; blood can back up and go the wrong way, causing the vein to puff up.

As a general surgery resident, operating on varicose veins was one of the first experiences I had of appearance-altering surgery. Although hardly the same as reducing a pair of EEs or removing pounds of skin off an arm, I found these small operations to be quite rewarding. And, as with many plastic surgeries, people can look *and* feel better afterward.

There are a few common causes of varicose veins:

1. **Heredity:** If your mom has varicose veins, then you are likely to develop them, too.

2. **Pregnancy:** The sudden added weight and other conditions in the body common with pregnancy can cause vein valves to malfunction, resulting in varicose veins, often for the first time.

3. **Standing for long periods:** If you are always on your feet, you are more likely to develop varicose veins. For this reason, certain jobs can predispose you to varicose veins, such as being a hairdresser or a surgeon (yikes for me!).

But you don't have to live with varicose veins. Fortunately, there are solutions, some more effective than others.

* **Elevate your legs:** Whenever you're at home, or even if possible at work, put your legs up above your heart. This decreases the pressure on your veins and can help the blood flow through the problem valves in the right direction. Although this doesn't solve your problem, it can help limit the severity of your varicose veins.

* **Compression hose or stockings:** It may sound "old lady" to you, but there are commercially available hose or stockings used by many hairdressers, surgeons, surgical technicians, and other people who stand all day. If you have a job where you stand for long periods (how about the security guard in a jewelry store?), even if you don't have varicose veins yet, using compression hose might help prevent varicose

veins from showing up. They don't look as "old lady" as they used to, and there are even fashionable compression stockings available online. One company, **Therafirm**, makes a garter-style thigh-high that can really get your man's attention! And they are available for men, too, so both of you can be fashionable and prevent varicose veins together. (How romantic.)

✳ **Endovenous laser therapy (EVT):** This is technically surgical but so minimally invasive that it doesn't feel like surgery. It is the newest treatment for varicose veins and is truly state-of-the-art, with minimal downtime and bleeding. If you really want to get rid of your varicose veins, this is what I recommend. For EVT, the surgeon inserts a laser fiber into the vein along its length. The laser is turned on and then slowly removed from the vein. As the laser is removed, this causes the blood in the vein to coagulate, and the vein collapses on itself. A similar procedure, which can be performed with a radiofrequency device instead of a laser, is called the **Venefit** procedure.

✳ **Surgical stripping:** This is the traditional treatment for varicose veins that I mentioned as one of the first operations I performed. The surgeon makes multiple small incisions on your legs and literally rips out the veins. This is quite invasive and results in permanent scars and a good amount of bleeding. For this reason, I generally don't recommend this method, as there is a much better and less traumatic option now.

Spider Veins

These are dark blue, black, or red squiggly veins that typically occur on the legs in clusters or streaks. As with varicose veins, they tend to increase with age, pregnancy, and jobs that require a lot of standing. They can also be genetic—some people develop them as teenagers but will likely accumulate more with every passing year. Unlike varicose veins, spider veins don't hurt and their treatment is purely cosmetic, but they tend to bother people quite a bit. Who wants legs that look like road maps? Like varicose veins, spider veins are caused by dysfunctional valves in the veins, causing the blood to back up and resulting in the veins looking dark but not swelling.

Over 50 percent of women have spider veins, including the most attractive women in Hollywood. I once did a segment on a short-lived talk show called *The Revolution*, where I discussed spider veins with my good friend, the beautiful (and current ABC News medical contributor and *The Doctors* co-host) Dr. Jennifer Ashton, where she revealed her spider veins on air. Nobody is immune, even some of the most glamorous women in Hollywood. Spider veins are certainly nothing to be ashamed of, but if they really bother you, they can be repaired.

* **Sclerotherapy:** The most common and effective treatment for spider veins, as for varicose veins, is slightly invasive, but unlike varicose vein treatment, the procedure to remove spider veins is very simple and relatively easy to undergo. It is called sclerotherapy. In this procedure, the plastic surgeon or dermatologist injects a **caustic solution** or **salt water** into the spider vein with a small needle. This causes the vein to close off and disappear. Often, one treatment is all that's needed for a dramatic improvement, but a second or even third treatment might be necessary. Sclerotherapy sounds easy and it is, but it also has some limitations. If the caustic sclerosant is accidentally injected outside the vein, it could cause damage to the surrounding tissues. This is a rare event, however. If the safer saltwater solution is used, there is a greater risk of the spider vein coming back, which could necessitate multiple treatments. Overall, I recommend saltwater injections if you want an inexpensive treatment. Sclerotherapy with actual sclerosing solution should ideally be saved for spider veins that are resistant to other treatments.

* **Laser treatment:** Instead of injecting the vein, laser treatments burn the blood vessel closed while leaving the skin unharmed. However, unlike sclerotherapy, laser treatments can involve four to six sessions for optimal effect. There is a risk of burns with almost any laser, and a risk of the vein coming back with time after this procedure. There are several lasers that target spider veins, but probably the most frequently used laser for this is an Nd:YAG laser, and it goes by the names **Cynosure Cynergy**, **Cutera Excel V**, and the **Candela GentleMax Pro**. Laser treatments are great for spider veins if you are needle-phobic and are willing and able to return for multiple treatments. Because it necessitates many sessions, however, the cost may be cumulatively higher than a single sclerotherapy session.

Caution!

Will vitamin K creams make your spider veins any better, as they claim? I'd love to tell you that applying a topical cream can improve the appearance of your spider veins. Unfortunately, there isn't any scientific evidence I know of that proves they work. I think it's a great idea to use vitamin K creams in addition to sclerotherapy or laser treatments, but as a stand-alone treatment, they will probably be very disappointing.

STRETCH MARKS

These permanent, accordionlike scars, otherwise known as striae, are caused by tearing of the deeper skin, or dermis, and people tend to really hate them. Stretch marks are typically associated with rapid growth (like the tummy of a pregnant woman or the thighs of a boy going through puberty) and rapid weight gain, so they are very common after pregnancy (those genetically predisposed are more likely to have a problem with them). I've even seen them, albeit rarely, in women who get breast implants. Their appearance is also affected by hormones, heredity, and medications.

So how do you get rid of stretch marks? Unfortunately, stretch marks are permanent. Short of cutting them out (such as with a tummy tuck), there is no permanent cure for stretch marks. There are, however, ways to reduce their appearance.

* **Laser treatments:** The first laser to be successfully used in treating stretch marks was the **pulsed dye laser** (**PDL**). A 2007 study published in *Dermatologic Surgery* revealed "good to very good" results in thirty-three out of thirty-seven patients.[33] The pulsed dye laser targets the red color of a newer stretch mark to reduce it and mildly thicken some of the collagen, making the stretch marks look closer in appearance to the normal skin around them. Typically, several treatments (four to six minimum) are necessary, and the procedure is virtually painless. We use the pulsed dye laser in my office, with some pretty dramatic improvements in stretch marks that are less than six months old. (It doesn't work as well for stretch marks that are years old.) The cost varies from $100 to $300 per treatment, and it can add up with the multiple treatments necessary. In 2010, the FDA approved the first **fractional laser** for use in improving the appearance of stretch marks. The **Palomar Lux 1540** is more aggressive than the pulsed dye laser, but it can reduce the appearance of stretch marks pretty impressively. I described how fractional lasers can tighten the collagen of the skin in chapter 3, and it works similarly when treating stretch marks. Basically, the stretch mark ends up smoother, tighter, and more similar to the surrounding skin. The drawback of this treatment is that it's expensive, with costs potentially in the thousands of dollars, and the skin typically requires several days or longer to heal. Although as of this writing the Lux 1540 is the only FDA-approved laser for stretch marks, you don't need to find a doctor with this exact laser. Most fractional lasers could probably be used to improve stretch marks in the same way.

* **Stretch mark creams:** There are several creams that claim to improve the appearance of stretch marks. Unfortunately, most of them won't give you a dramatic

improvement. It's just impossible for most creams to affect the deeper skin (dermis) tears of stretch marks enough to make a major change in how they look. The one cream worth trying for improving stretch marks, however, is a retinol cream, or better yet, tretinoin. Because it is scientifically proven to thicken the dermis, tretinoin is your best shot at improving the appearance of stretch marks without lasers or surgery. Be careful with it, though, since the skin of your body may be more sensitive to tretinoin than the skin of your face. It's probably best to start with a milder retinol cream and progress to tretinoin as your tolerance increases. Because of the potential sensitivities, it's probably best to treat your stretch marks with tretinoin only under the care of a dermatologist or plastic surgeon.

* **Prevention:** The best way to noninvasively treat a stretch mark is to prevent it from appearing. Keep in mind, however, that if you are genetically predisposed to stretch marks, you may get them no matter what you do. There is no way to prove that people who used the following strategies and didn't get stretch marks *would have* gotten them had they not tried these, so while they can't hurt, know that they might not help, either:

  ▶ **Moisturizers:** Our moms are always right. I instruct all my pregnant patients to liberally apply moisturizer to their tummies throughout their pregnancies. Cocoa butter is probably as good as any. The idea is that dry skin may be more prone to tearing than supple, moisturized skin. There is no science to prove it, but decades upon decades of moms swear by their cocoa butter. That's good enough for me!

  ▶ **Omega-3 fatty acids:** We covered these fatty acids and how they can make our skin age more slowly and even look younger in chapter 5, but their moisturizing effects and positive impact on skin elasticity can also theoretically help prevent stretch marks from forming. Some foods that are high in omega-3 fatty acids include fish, walnuts, and flaxseed. If you are pregnant, make sure to discuss a safe amount of fish in your diet with your obstetrician.

SCARS

Fact of life: Scars are permanent, and the longer you live, the more likely you're going to have a few. We may be able to erase mental or psychological scars (although not easily!), but physical scars, such as we get from surgery and traumatic accidents, are for life. No matter how good a surgeon is, what cream you put on the scar afterward, or what laser treatment is used on the scar, it will never completely disappear.

In fact, it may surprise you to know that the amount of control a surgeon has over the final appearance of a scar is pretty darn tiny. I tell my patients that what I can do during a two- or three-hour operation to make your scar look good pales in comparison to what your body will do to mature your scar, twenty-four hours a day, seven days a week, four weeks a month, for six to twenty-four months—the time required for a scar to completely mature. I have a lot of patients credit me for their almost imperceptible, "invisible" scars after surgery, and as much as I'd like to take the credit, that would mean taking the blame when the scar doesn't heal as well as we'd like. As a plastic surgeon I can prevent a scar from having small suture tracks around it (a result of leaving the stitches in too long), from looking jagged or uneven, or from being placed in a bad location. I can't 100 percent prevent it from thickening or widening, however. Your body determines how that will happen. That being said, there are some things we can do to improve the chances your scar will heal well or look better than it currently does.

Keloid Scars and Hypertrophic Scars

Two types of scars can result from overgrowth of collagen and therefore scar tissue. Hypertrophic scars are thick and raised but still exist within the original cut or incision. Keloids are hypertrophic scars that have grown so thick that they, by definition, extend beyond the borders of the initial scar, and sometimes they can be painful or itchy. Hypertrophic scars and keloids may form because of a genetic propensity, and they are also most common in younger people and in people with darker skin. Any scar could potentially become a hypertrophic scar or a keloid, but many scars do not. Scars on certain parts of the body are at higher risk of becoming keloids. These areas include the middle of the chest, the shoulders and knees, the upper back, and, strangely enough, the earlobes. There is no 100 percent guaranteed way to reduce, eliminate, or prevent a keloid or hypertrophic scar, but there are a handful of things you can try that can help. Typically keloids or thicker scars are treated least invasively at first, and then if these treatments don't work, you progress to more aggressive options. Let's look at treatments in that order.

* **Vitamin E:** The easiest, least expensive way to reduce the risk of a scar becoming thick is to apply vitamin E to a new scar. Vitamin E is a potent antioxidant that some people believe can help prevent scars from thickening. You can purchase vitamin E capsules at pharmacies and health-food stores. Break the capsule open and apply to the scar twice a day. If your skin becomes irritated, though, discontinue the treatment, as the science supporting vitamin E in helping prevent keloid scars is minimal and not worth suffering side effects.

* **Occlusion:** Some plastic surgeons believe that the act of occluding a scar (keeping it covered with slight pressure and avoiding exposure to air) can prevent it from becoming thick and keloidal. The exact mechanism for how this works is unknown, but it has led some plastic surgeons to recommend taping scars for long periods of time. You can easily do this at home by purchasing some paper medical tape and applying it over your scars. Change the tape when it gets gross (typically after a couple of days). As long as your skin isn't reacting to the adhesive on the tape, then you can continue taping the scars for several weeks or even several months. Another way to occlude the scars is to apply petroleum jelly. Some plastic surgeons believe that keeping the scars moist and occluded with petroleum jelly can be just as effective as more expensive scar creams. For earlobe keloids, which are more common among African Americans, there are specialized earrings that put pressure over the scar to prevent it from becoming a keloid. These can be purchased online and come in many shapes and styles.

* **Scar cream:** If you are okay with spending a little more money, commercial-grade scar creams and products are probably a better bet to reduce your risk of a thick scar than either vitamin E or occlusion. Scientific studies show that silicone-based scar creams and silicone sheeting (rubberlike adhesive sheets that stick to the scars) are effective in reducing the risk of thick scars and even thinning out currently thick scars. Whether you use silicone creams or sheets, a 2009 study showed it probably doesn't matter.[34] Currently I prefer **Silagen**, a 100 percent pure silicone gel that dries into a protective barrier over the scar, helping to hydrate, flatten, and soften it. It appears to be the best of both worlds, as it applies like a cream but leaves an adhesive patch like silicone sheeting, lasting several hours. **BioCorneum** is similar to Silagen but contains sunblock, which can be very helpful in sun-exposed areas. Scar creams can be expensive, though, ranging from $50 to $125 for a tube that lasts a couple of months. Silicone sheeting can cost significantly more.

* **Laser treatment:** If topical treatments aren't working and your scar is getting thicker or isn't improving, then the next step is to try laser treatments. Studies have shown that a **pulsed dye laser** (**PDL**) can be effective in reducing the redness of a scar and sometimes decreasing the size of a scar. We typically recommend once-a-month PDL treatments for thick and/or red scars. It can take six to twelve months or more for optimal improvement. If you have a keloid, some insurances may cover laser treatments. Check with your insurance company to see. The laser treatments typically have no downtime and are virtually painless, but they may leave behind some temporary bruising.

✳ **Steroid injection:** If you're trying lasers and topicals without improvement, or if the scar has become a bona fide large keloid, then the next step is injection of a steroid. When a steroid is injected into a thick scar, it can help break down the excessive collagen buildup, causing the scar to get thinner. An added bonus: Symptoms like itching and pain are often relieved with steroid injections. Steroid injections aren't without their potential risks, though. My patients often ask whether, as with anabolic steroids, steroid injections could make the testicles shrink. Not to worry—they won't have this particular effect. However, they can shrink the thickness of the normal skin around the keloid. This can result in an undesirable, permanent indentation to the normal skin surrounding the keloid. Because of this, I restrict steroid injections to those keloids and thick scars that won't respond to lasers and topicals.

✳ **Surgery:** If all else fails, then keloids can be cut out and the skin resutured. Unfortunately, keloids have a high rate of recurrence, so reoperating on the area is something I do as a last resort. In many cases, the new scar forms another keloid. Plus, every time the keloid is cut out, the scar gets just a little longer.

✳ **Radiation:** The only other option for keloid treatment is radiation. Radiation is reserved for keloids that are resistant to all the other therapies and must be reduced for a medical reason, such as pain, itching, and major deformity. (This is a last-case scenario, because we all want to minimize our exposure to radiation over a lifetime.) The protocol typically requires anywhere from one to three radiotherapy treatments following surgical removal of the keloid, and can be effective for even the most stubborn keloids.[35]

Acne Scars

Acne scarring is one of the most difficult cosmetic skin issues to treat. So many people have suffered through teenage acne, leaving both psychological and physical scars. My father-in-law, Jim, suffered from terrible acne as a teenager. He was so embarrassed to suffer ridicule with names like "Pizza Face" that he spent most of his adolescence alone in his room, listening to music and dreaming of having a different face. He continues, to this day, to feel self-conscious about his acne scars.

The best treatment for acne scarring is, obviously, not to develop it in the first place. The good news is that today kids shouldn't be forced to suffer through acne problems like in Jim's day, when the treatments were pretty rudimentary and ineffective at treating cystic acne. Benzoyl peroxide, tretinoin, blue light treatments, and isotretinoin have improved the lives of millions of teens and even adults.

The treatments for acne scarring have also improved, but unfortunately there is no magic bullet for acne scars. There is no way to make them completely disappear and give you skin as smooth as if you never had acne in the first place. However, there have been and continue to be a plethora of treatments that have proven effective in reducing the appearance of acne scars. First, a few that don't work so well, just so you know about them:

* **Dermabrasion:** Decades ago Jim had his whole face dermabraded. During this treatment a doctor takes a diamond-tipped burr and literally sands the upper layer of skin off your face. Although still used for small areas (I like to use it to reduce the wrinkles of the upper lip), today it's considered obsolete for large areas like the whole face. The problem with dermabrading acne scars is that any effective acne treatment must reach all the way down to the deeper skin, or dermis, for visible results. This leaves the face covered in blood and takes weeks to heal. Yes, you may walk out of the procedure with a crimson mask of blood. Yuck! For this reason, I don't recommend this.

* **Ablative lasers:** Once ablative lasers were introduced in the 1990s, they became the treatment of choice for acne scarring. The problem with the older ablative lasers, like the CO_2 laser, was the weeks of pain and downtime that resulted and the many potential complications, such as permanent lightening of the skin. However, the results in improving acne scars were impressive.

Today, all the treatments to improve acne scarring are aimed at getting results similar to those of the old ablative CO_2 lasers, but without the drawbacks. These treatments, such as surgery (cutting out each individual scar), lasers (like fractional lasers and picosecond lasers), and radiofrequency devices (like eMatrix and Fractora), can have pretty impressive results, but they can be very expensive, costing in the thousands of dollars. However, if you want to improve your acne scars and spend as little as possible, check out my two suggestions below.

* **Chemical peels:** Chemical peels improve acne scarring by exfoliating the superficial skin (epidermis) and tightening up the deeper skin (dermis). Keep in mind that the aggressiveness of the peel is directly proportional to the amount of improvement you will get. And your best results will occur with a regimen of several deeper peels, not just one. Although there are a lot of chemical peels to choose from, such as the **Obagi Blue Peel, ZO Controlled Depth Peel, VI Peel, TCA Peel, Phenol Peel, Jessner's Peel**, and dozens of others, you will see improvement in acne scarring only if the peel's effects extend to the dermis. In general, this will require at least a couple of

days' downtime after the treatment, if not a full week. Lunchtime peels or at-home peels, which typically treat only the epidermis, will not improve your acne scarring. They just don't go deep enough. If you're considering having a series of chemical peels to improve your acne scarring, make sure to discuss with your doctor about just how deep the peels will go, and how long your recovery time will be. The peels should extend at least into the superficial dermis and give you a few days of peeling, minimum. Anything less than that will be a waste of time and money.

* **Microneedling:** This is a newer treatment that is being used more and more for acne scarring. During this procedure, a practitioner uses several tiny needles (with either a roller or a handheld motorized device) to puncture the skin down to the dermis to encourage collagen stimulation. Afterward, the practitioner applies growth factors to the treated skin as a way to get the growth factors to seep into the deeper layers of the skin. The growth factors can take the form of a serum (such as **Tensage**) or even your own blood (which is filled with growth factors). The downtime is typically a day or two, and the treatment must be repeated several times for optimal results. Microneedling is a lot less expensive than laser treatments and has less downtime than chemical peels, making it a valid option for many people who either can't afford laser treatments or don't have the time to peel for a week. One study reported a 50–75 percent improvement in the appearance of acne scars after five treatments.[36] Not bad! If you suffer from acne scarring and you've believed that there isn't a solution, microneedling is something to strongly consider. It's relatively inexpensive, it's effective, and you can get some nice improvement if you stick with it.

> ## Warning!
>
> If you have a history of cold sores, make sure to tell your doctor before having microneedling, chemical peels, or laser treatments. Even if your last cold sore was ten years ago, you'll be at risk of a breakout after one of these procedures. Rest assured, you can still have the treatment, though, as long as your doctor puts you on an antiviral (like Valtrex) before, during, and after you have it done.

HAIRY ISSUES

As you age, your hair changes. You may start growing hair in places you never grew it before (and never wanted to—hello, chin hair!). The hair you want to keep thick and luxurious begins to get thinner and sparser (in both men and women). And of course, graying. For most people, shaving or waxing, the occasional plucking, and, of course, the monthly visit to the salon to keep the gray roots at bay are usually enough. These procedures are relatively easy, are inexpensive, and don't have many risks. However, if your hair issues go beyond what you are willing or able to achieve with shaving or waxing, or if you are just sick of shaving or waxing, you can take hair removal to the next level with more permanent solutions.

* **Laser hair removal:** Hair removal lasers have been in use since 1997. Virtually every major cosmetic laser company has a laser hair removal device. The treatments are well tolerated, feel like a rubber band snapping at your skin, and can blast away hair follicles. The most common areas for hair removal on women are the underarms and bikini area, but it can also treat unwanted dark facial hair that begins to appear with age. In men, whose body hair can get more profuse just as head hair is disappearing, the back is most commonly treated. Typically, laser hair removal necessitates multiple treatments. As hair growth slows and hair thins, most people find that they need to come back for treatments only every few years. The technology really hasn't changed a lot over the years, but the newer machines are able to get rid of hair quicker, in less time and with fewer treatments. The cost varies quite a bit depending on the size of the area being treated and the number of treatments needed. Most people need at least six to eight treatments for optimal results, and each treatment can range in price from $100 to $500, or even more (if the person has her arms, legs, and bikini areas done all at once). I recommend laser hair removal as the best option for getting rid of hair permanently.

Caution!

Two cautions about laser hair removal:

1. Laser hair removal does not work for blond, white, or gray hair, because the laser targets the color of the hair follicle. People with light hair might consider electrolysis instead.

2. People with darker skin should be very choosy about the laser that is used for their hair removal. Not all lasers work for darker skin, as some have a much higher risk for burns. Currently, one of the best devices for laser hair removal in darker skin is the 1064 nm Nd:YAG laser, which goes by names such as the **Sciton ClearScan YAG**, the **Cutera excel HR**, and the **Cynosure Elite**, among others.

* **Electrolysis:** Electrolysis is a valid alternative for people who have hair that won't be affected by laser hair removal. In this procedure, a very fine needle is inserted into the hair follicle and delivers an electrical current to destroy the part of the hair follicle

that causes the hair to grow. The hair is then removed and doesn't usually grow back. The great thing about electrolysis is that it can be used on hair of any color, including gray, white, and blond. It's not my first choice for permanent hair reduction in people with darker hair, though, because it usually requires upward of ten to fifteen treatments for maximal effect (compared to six to eight treatments for laser hair removal), and it can be a long, somewhat excruciating process. Also unlike laser hair removal, which can treat several hair follicles with each laser pulse, each hair must be treated individually. This can take quite a long time if you are treating large areas of the body. For this reason, I recommend electrolysis if you are Caucasian with blond, gray, or white hair that you'd like to permanently remove from your eyebrows, upper lip, or chin. Otherwise, go for the laser treatment.

Insider Tip

Treating the bikini lines is one thing, but I strongly discourage women from doing permanent Brazilian (completely bare) bikini laser hair removal. It's a good idea to keep at least some hair down there, because it can help to prevent infections in the genital region. In fact, the incidence of bacterial vaginitis is higher in women with Brazilian bikini waxes than in women with some pubic hair present. Also, styles change. Just because completely bald genitals are popular now doesn't mean that they will be popular ten years from now. There are even recent reports of people undergoing pubic hair transplants in Korea and Japan! I suggest keeping at least some of what nature gave you.

* **At-home hair removal systems:** There are a handful of home laser hair removal devices on the market today. Typically they cost several hundred dollars and the results aren't quite as dramatic as laser hair removal done in the office. Home laser hair removal devices utilize pulsed light to destroy hair follicles, can take thirty to sixty minutes for each treatment session, and take six to eight treatments for maximal results. Of these devices, my favorite is the **Silk'n Flash&Go**, an ✳ AGE FIX FAVORITE . **The Tria Hair Removal Laser 4X** is another popular option, but it costs over twice as much as the Silk'n version. Both can be bought online and should not be used on people with darker skin. My main issue with at-home laser hair removal is that the treatments can be pretty tedious. The spot size (treatment area) is quite small, so if you are treating larger areas like your legs, it can take a long time to perform each individual treatment. However, if you want to save some money and don't mind doing it yourself, then at-home laser hair removal can be a reasonable option for you.

THINNING HAIR

Our society isn't kind to us regarding our hair. Women are expected to have a full head of luxurious hair, but be completely bald everywhere else. Men, too, are expected to have a full head of hair, but back hair? Eww. Although celebrities like Andre Agassi, Bruce Willis, and Dwayne "the Rock" Johnson have shown us that bald can be beautiful, the majority of hair loss remedies are developed, packaged, and marketed toward men. With one major exception (Propecia), these treatments can also be used on women. People don't often think about women going bald, because it doesn't usually happen as obviously as in men, but many older women notice extreme thinning, even patches where the scalp is visible. Hair loss and thinning can make everyone feel older than their years.

Before we get to the treatment options for hair loss, we should at least touch on the causes, since the cause can be even more important than the solution. Hair loss can be stress related, in which case the solution is to seek ways to reduce your stress. It can be related to medical conditions such as hypothyroidism, anemia, lupus, and polycystic ovarian syndrome (PCOS), necessitating blood tests to determine potential treatments. It can also be due to a genetic condition called androgenic alopecia. There are so many causes for thinning hair that I encourage you to consult with a physician (typically a board-certified dermatologist) who specializes in hair loss prior to undergoing any treatment. With thinning hair, the treatment is always determined by the cause.

Here are my recommendations for treating thinning hair, in the order that I recommend you try them:

* **Reduce stress.** It's widely known that stress can precipitate hair loss, a temporary phenomenon called telogen effluvium. Working with a therapist to reduce stress is a great way to combat this.

* **Increase your protein intake.** Protein forms the building blocks of healthy hair. Focus on healthy protein sources like nuts, beans, and lean meats.

* **Supplements, such as biotin and zinc,** have been touted for improving hair growth but probably will not be helpful unless your doctor determines you have a deficiency.

* **Minoxidil 2% (Rogaine)** is the only topical medication approved by the FDA for female-pattern hair loss and should be the first medical treatment that you try. Men can use a higher strength (5%) and combine this with **finasteride (Propecia)**.

If you are female, do not try 5% minoxidil or finasteride unless your doctor recommends it, since you may develop some undesired side effects (bearded lady, anyone?).

* **Low-light laser therapy** is an option if you're female and minoxidil isn't working for you. This is currently all the rage in treating hair loss, and it goes by the names **HairMax LaserComb**, **iGrow laser helmet**, and the **LaserCap**. These are considered "cold" lasers that can painlessly and noninvasively stimulate hair growth. Many studies have shown low-light laser therapy to be effective in treating thinning hair, but these devices can be costly, starting at $300 and up.

* **Platelet-rich plasma (PRP) with microneedling**, used in combination, is the newest treatment for thinning hair. PRP is obtained by taking a sample of your own blood, spinning it in a centrifuge, and isolating the plasma, which is rich in growth factors. These growth factors are believed to stimulate hair growth, and they penetrate to the deeper skin via the small channels (holes) created by microneedling. The jury is still out on this one, but many of my colleagues have been quite impressed with the results. This is an invasive procedure, however, and can cost $500 or more. Therefore, I recommend trying this only if the above treatments aren't successful in thickening your hair.

* **Follicular unit extraction (FUE) with the NeoGraft** device is the newest state-of-the-art hair transplant system. With all the nonsurgical options for thinning hair, surgery shouldn't be necessary unless you have actual bald areas, where there is no hair growing, and you can't live with it. If that's the case, then hair transplants may be your only real option. Gone are the days when plastic surgeons would perform hair plugs, making your hair look like a cheap doll's hair. This high-tech system creates almost no visible scars in either the donor site or the recipient site (the place where the hair is grafted to). If you need actual hair replacement, then make sure your doctor uses the FUE technique!

ODOR ISSUES

It's something nobody wants to hear: "You stink." Even if nobody says it, what if they are thinking it? Bad breath and body odor are two very common situations that most people hope to avoid. Although teenagers are notoriously stinky, body odor issues usually abate after adolescence. However, in some people they can return with age, as hormones go haywire again and dental problems may increase. For others, BO and bad breath are a lifelong issue. Sure, bad breath and BO don't necessarily make you look older (actually, if people are standing farther away from you, your wrinkles will be less noticeable!), but they can make you feel older, or at least worse about how you come across to the world. However, knowing your breath is fresh and you smell good will certainly make you feel more confident, and that could be worth a shopping cart full of antiaging creams.

If you do struggle with odor issues, you will be happy to know there are real solutions. Let's get you smelling sweeter.

Bad Breath

Bad breath is extremely common. More than 50 million people suffer from chronic halitosis (bad breath) in the United States. Contrary to popular belief, bad breath is not caused by cavities, gum disease, or not brushing your teeth. Very rarely, bad breath can be caused by a real medical problem, but 95 percent of the time, it is simply a side effect of sulfur-causing bacteria accumulating on the back of your tongue.

This might sound like something you could brush away or flush away, but toothbrushes don't reach far enough back on the tongue, and mouthwashes only mask the problem. However, there is a solution that can cure 99 percent of bad breath issues.

* **ProFresh:** The ProFresh system is available for anyone to purchase, but it is essentially a medical solution for bad breath. It is the only system that uses active chlorine dioxide, the most effective ingredient to kill sulfur-producing bacteria on the back of the tongue and neutralize the sulfur smell. Use it for two minutes twice a day and use the tongue scraper that comes with the kit. Tongue scraping is one of the most important aspects of treating bad breath. The ProFresh system comes with a great tongue scraper that can reach places your toothbrush can't. The Starter Kit is available online for about $40.

* **Tongue scraper and baking soda:** If you want the most effective part of the ProFresh system without the price tag, then buy a tongue scraper separately and use it every day to help remove the stinky little critters from the back of your tongue. If you pair this with a regimen of brushing your teeth with baking soda, this will give you the benefit of additional odor removal and will even gradually whiten your teeth. But don't just brush your teeth—brush the sides of your mouth, all over your gums, the roof of your mouth, the tip and bottom side of your tongue, and as far back on your tongue as you can reach without gagging.

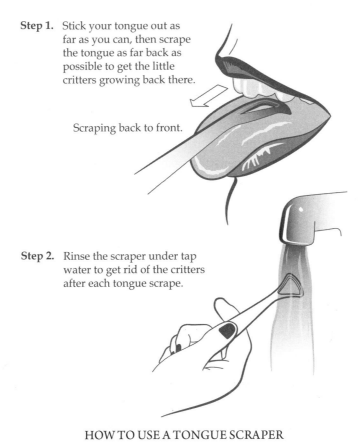

Step 1. Stick your tongue out as far as you can, then scrape the tongue as far back as possible to get the little critters growing back there.

Scraping back to front.

Step 2. Rinse the scraper under tap water to get rid of the critters after each tongue scrape.

HOW TO USE A TONGUE SCRAPER

Some more breath-freshening and odor-reducing secrets:

❋ **Don't eat that.** It's not really a secret that certain foods make your breath stink more than others. If you have a problem with bad breath, avoid foods like garlic and onions, which can increase the risk of halitosis and increase the sulfur smell emanating from your mouth.

❋ **Don't drink/smoke that.** Coffee breath isn't the nicest thing to get in the face, either, and neither is beer breath. Obviously, smoking can make your breath smell pretty bad. (Just one more reason to quit.)

❋ **Chew cinnamon gum or any sugarless gum.** Chewing gum not only helps clean your teeth of bacteria but keeps saliva production going, which rinses out your mouth with its natural antibacterial properties.

* **Eat more high-fiber foods.** High-fiber foods encourage the production of saliva to begin the digestive process while chewing. Saliva not only has natural antibacterial elements in it but keeps your mouth moist. A dry mouth tends to be stinkier.

* **Eat more raw, crunchy fruits and veggies.** Not only do these help scrape your teeth clean, but the enzymes they contain can have a breath-freshening effect. Especially try apples, celery, and carrots.

* **Nosh on fresh parsley or mint leaves.** These fresh herbs not only contain antibacterial elements but are full of chlorophyll, which is a natural detoxifying agent. I never understood why the chopped steaks I used to eat at Ponderosa as a teenager always came with a little parsley sprig as a garnish. Now I know the truth: It was to help prevent the dreaded "dragon breath."

* **Try fennel seeds.** Chew a few after every meal. These are also supposed to improve breath odor. You may notice that Indian restaurants sometimes have a bowl at the counter where other restaurants might keep a jar of mints. They are to counteract the chicken tikka masala you just ate!

* **Drink plenty of water.** Not only will this help flush out the bacteria from your mouth, but it will also keep your mouth from drying out and creating unpleasant odors.

* **Clean your dentures.** If you have them, keep them squeaky clean. Old, dirty dentures are a common cause of bad breath.

Beauty Secret

Can you guess the first thing I notice when meeting someone new? Since I'm a plastic surgeon, you may think it's the person's nose, neck, or facial wrinkles. Nope! It's the color of their teeth! Yellowing teeth can convey many things about us, whether true or not, such as poor oral hygiene, smoking, and age. Dentists have made billions on expensive teeth-whitening treatments, such as trays and lasers. But you don't need them! Here's a simple tip that can help dramatically whiten your teeth without paying hundreds or thousands on expensive treatments. Try **Crest 3D White whitening toothpaste**, an ✳ AGE FIX FAVORITE .

Now, I know you've probably tried other whitening toothpastes and have been disappointed at their lack of results, but this whitening toothpaste is different. It actually works. Try it for two weeks, and if you haven't seen the changes you are looking for, then add the **Crest 3D White Glamorous White Rinse** for an extra whitening effect. Both of these products should cost you less than $7 each at the drugstore. I think you'll be pleasantly surprised. I've been using Crest 3D whitening toothpaste for a couple of years now and have ditched my whitening trays altogether.

Body Odor

The only odor issue worse than bad breath is BO. Maybe you've been stuck in an elevator or on a train with somebody who reeked. It's not a pleasant experience, and most people don't want to be that person everyone moves away from, but some people really can't help it. Body odor is most often caused by a combination of perspiration and bacteria, and some people are simply more prone to sweating and accumulating bacteria on the skin. The trick is to tackle both of these culprits at the same time. Here are some good options:

* **miraDry:** This product is an FDA-approved device for permanently reducing excessive armpit sweating. Although not FDA-approved for odor reduction yet, it also appears to be very effective for reducing smelly armpits. It dries the armpits out by destroying the sweat glands. Combine the miraDry with some good antibacterial soap, and your armpit stink is a thing of the past! For more on the wonders of miraDry, which I consider to be another one of my ✳ AGE FIX FAVORITES , check out the next section in this chapter, which covers what to do about excessive sweating.

* **Apple cider vinegar or lemon juice:** Wouldn't vinegar in your armpits make the smell worse? Surprisingly, no. Apple cider vinegar lowers the pH of your skin, killing off odor-causing bacteria. You could also try lemon juice. For either, apply to your armpits with a cotton ball every morning. However, avoid open cuts or sores, and don't apply right after shaving your armpits. That would sting!

* **Milk of magnesia:** Although it's typically used as a constipation remedy, some people claim to have had great improvement in odor issues when applying milk of magnesia to the armpits.

Keep in mind that none of the above remedies constitute an antiperspirant. Sweating is a different issue (covered in the next section).

But what about the rest of your bod? We all know that people can stink in places beyond their armpits. To decrease overall body odor, remember that sweat plus bacteria equals stink. You may need to shower more often than people who don't have body odor issues to keep the bacteria off. Also take a look at your diet. I suggest making these two simple changes:

* **Eat more chlorophyll-rich foods.** Chlorophyll is a natural detoxifying agent of the body. Therefore, eating chlorophyll-rich foods can help with the elimination of smelly toxins. Foods rich in chlorophyll are leafy, green vegetables, like spinach, kale, broccoli, and lettuce. Yep, a big daily salad could keep you smelling fresher!

* **Take acidophilus pills or eat more yogurt (or both).** Acidophilus and other probiotic bacteria help balance the bacterial content in the digestive tract. Help your gut bacteria work in your favor.

* **Sweat less.** Read on!

EXCESSIVE SWEATING

Sure, you drip at the gym or on your daily run, but if you've got sweat dripping from your underarms or sliding down your cleavage when you're just sitting at the office, or if you frequently have to change your shirt because you sweat through it every day, then you probably have an issue with excessive sweating. It's estimated that over 50 million Americans, or one in five, suffer from excessive sweating, usually of the armpits. Can you do something about this? Absolutely!

In the past, neurosurgeons performed invasive surgeries to cut the nerves that led to areas of excess sweating. This was the only surgical option for major sweaters while I was in residency training. With the newest advances in nonsurgical sweat reduction, however, I don't hear of these surgeries being performed much anymore. That's good news for everyone. Instead, you've got a few much less invasive options.

Botox

Botox injections are very effective in temporarily reducing excess sweating. Botox acts by blocking signals to the nerves that create sweat. Botox can be injected into many areas where sweating is excessive, including the armpits, palms, and soles of the feet. It takes about a week to work, and it lasts approximately six months. The only problem is that the results aren't permanent, and Botox is expensive. The cost of injecting the armpits can run over $1,000. However, for areas other than the armpits, Botox is still the gold standard for excessive sweating.

miraDry

For the armpits, we have a game changer. It's the **✳ AGE FIX FAVORITE** I mentioned earlier in this chapter, and it's a treatment called miraDry. This treatment is available only from doctors, but it really works. It utilizes microwave technology to reduce sweating on average 82 percent after two treatments! The miraDry treatments can be painful, so local anesthetics are injected to numb up the armpit. This makes the procedure virtually painless. The treatment takes about an hour, and most patients have some swelling and redness of the armpits for several days afterward. The discomfort is mild, though, and typically very tolerable with just over-the-counter pain medications like Motrin.

I recently purchased this machine because I was so impressed by its results. Most lasers and similar technology take multiple treatments to see any improvement. I've seen so many people who've had immediate and lasting results with miraDry that I think it'll be the gold standard for sweat reduction of the armpits for many, many years to come. One of my miraDry patients complained before the treatment that she had to wear a sleeveless wedding dress to avoid armpit sweat stains. After her series of two treatments she sent me a photo of her at the Grand Canyon in hundred-degree weather wearing a short-sleeved T-shirt with completely dry armpits!

Another benefit of miraDry is that it can also improve the smell caused by sweaty armpits. Although the device is FDA-approved only for treatment of the armpits, my hope is that the device can be made more versatile to treat sweating of other areas, such as the hands and feet. It's not cheap, but if excessive sweating is ruining your life, it may be the best money you'll ever spend on a medical treatment. A miraDry treatment costs about $1,500, and most people typically need two treatments.

AGING HANDS AND FEET

Your face can look great. Your hair can look fantastic. Your curves can look bangin'. And then…you notice your hands and feet. I've seen websites that feature "hot celebrities with disgusting feet" or that highlight a beautiful but aging actress's hands, with text about how old they look. This is a rude and exploitive thing to do to anyone, but it also highlights a perhaps unfortunate fact of our current culture: If you are trying to look younger, your hands and feet can quickly give you away.

Younger Hands

Our hands show our age more than any other part of our bodies. People may not look at your hands before they look at your face, but when they do look, what story will your hands tell? The hands are so often untended and abused. Unlike the face and neck, we forget about them. On top of this neglect, hands are constantly subjected to agents that dry them out (water and dishwashing soap, cleaning products), UV rays (especially your left hand on the steering wheel), and extreme temperatures (like frigid cold temps in northern states). Yet, many women who constantly put creams and potions on their faces and necks might remember to moisturize their hands once or twice a day at most.

This is why, as we get older, the skin of our hands dries out. But aging does more to our hands than dry them out. It also thins them out. The soft, fatty layer that covers youthful hands disappears and we begin to see the tendons and veins underneath the thin, sun-spotted skin.

If you wish your hands looked a decade younger (to match your age-defying face!), then you have options.

Celeb Spot

A good example of a celebrity with aging hands is Madonna. She is now in her fifties, and her face remains without wrinkles and with tight, smooth skin. Her cheeks are plump and soft. Yet, this is all in stark contrast to her incredibly lean physique and her hands, which have lost volume over the years and look bony–certainly older than her face. There isn't necessarily anything wrong with this. We use our hands throughout our lives, and it is only natural that they will show some wear and tear. Also, the hands lose volume with age. This happens to many women in their fifties. One day they look down and wonder, "What happened to my hands?" They can look more sinewy with more prominent veins, and the skin can get crepey or wrinkly. Madonna might not mind her hands at all, and you might not mind yours, either, but I do have patients who come to me to fix this exact problem.

FAT GRAFTING / TRANSFER

One of the major aging changes to the hands is loss of subcutaneous fat, or fat underneath the skin's surface. This exposes veins and tendons that nobody sees in the hands of teenagers. There is one surgical technique to reverse this, and it is called fat grafting or transfer. This technique sucks fat from one part of the body with a big needle and injects it into the hands. As with fat grafts to the cheeks, not all of the fat stays put, but a portion (typically about half) stays long-term, causing the backs of your hands to look softer and less bony. The surgery takes an hour or two and costs approximately $4,000. This procedure is considered by many plastic surgeons as the current gold standard for hand rejuvenation, but this is not something I do. I was scared away from it by a patient I saw many years ago. She was a woman who was obviously a plastic surgery addict. Of course I didn't say it out loud to her, but when I saw her, all I could think was that her face looked completely plastic. Her lips and cheeks were overly plumped, her eyebrows were overly arched, her skin was as smooth and white as porcelain, and her neck looked impossibly tight. I couldn't believe someone had done this to her. She came to see me in consultation to fix up her hands because her last plastic surgeon tried to inject fat into both of her hands, but ran out of fat once he finished with her left one. So her left hand was plump and actually kind of lumpy-looking, while her right hand was thin and veiny. Not the look anybody would want! I referred her to a hand-fat-grafting specialist in New York but otherwise recommended procedures to actually reverse the work she'd had done.

SCULPTRA

Sculptra is a long-acting injectable volumizer that some doctors are using to thicken skin and add volume to thinning hands. Basically, it's a liquid that is injected into areas that need plumping up. The Sculptra interacts with the soft tissues in the area to create new collagen and gradually plumps the area. Its results appear slowly and usually take at least three treatments for maximal effect. The results last approximately two years, maybe more. Keep in mind that this is an off-label treatment, as the FDA has not approved Sculptra for use in the hands. However, I do believe it is a reasonable treatment to have performed if you want your hands to look plumper without surgery. Each treatment costs $500–$1,000.

MOISTURIZE

If you'd rather keep the needles away from your hands and you can handle the thinning but not the aging skin, then you have a lot more affordable and noninvasive options. Job one: Moisturize. Moisturizing is the most important thing you can do to rejuvenate your hands at home. As I've already mentioned, our hands take tons of abuse and get dried out all day long. Doctors and nurses, for example, wash their hands countless times per day. We wash dishes, we forget to wear our gloves on a cold day, we garden, we clean things. This isn't just an issue for women, either. I once did a local TV segment on dry skin in the winter and brought a couple of good hand creams with me. I was swarmed not by women, but by men! The cameramen, producers, directors, and production assistants all showed me their cracked, dry, bleeding hands and asked me what they could do about them.

If you want to get serious about moisturizing your hands, I strongly recommend that you buy two kinds of moisturizers, one to use during the day and one to use at night:

Your Day Hand Moisturizer: A moisturizer for the day needs to pass the doorknob test. It passes this test if, after applying it to your hands, you can turn a doorknob without your hand slipping all over it. Most daytime moisturizers are good humectants, meaning they retain moisture in the skin. These often contain glycerin as the major ingredient. I highly recommend **Eucerin Intensive Repair Extra-Enriched Hand Creme**. You can purchase it at most drugstores, and it typically costs less than $7. This cream feels awesome on your hands. It's thick enough to provide great hydration but leaves a very thin film that is neither tacky nor too slippery. It passes the doorknob test with flying colors. Keep a tube of this in your purse or in your desk drawer and apply several times a day. Even in the coldest, driest climates it will keep your hands nice and soft.

Your Night Hand Moisturizer: Hand moisturizers for use at night are typically more occlusive, or thick. Because you don't need to be turning handles or shaking hands at night, it's perfectly fine to apply a thicker layer of a heavier moisturizer to restore and soothe your hands at night. I highly recommend **Neutrogena Norwegian Formula Hand Cream**, an ✺ AGE FIX FAVORITE . It's fragrance free, and a perfect combination of humectant and occlusive. It's thicker than the Eucerin Intensive Repair hand cream, but can be used in a larger amount at night or a smaller amount during the day. It also passes the doorknob test. This cream is also typically less than $6 or $7.

If your hands are extremely dry, cracked, or even bleeding, then try **Burt's Bees Almond Milk Beeswax Hand Crème**. This occlusive moisturizer is more of a paste than a cream, and it contains almond milk and beeswax, in addition to the humectant glycerin. It really locks the moisture into your hands and is great for night use. Plus, it smells tasty.

Just three more tips to maximize your hand-moisturizing efforts:

1. In addition to morning and evening, always apply moisturizer after washing and towel drying, when your hands are still a little damp. The moisturizer can lock in the moisture and prevent your hands from ever drying out. Then apply a pair of cotton gloves after moisturizing in the evening. The gloves can lock in the moisture to your hands overnight. When you wake up the next morning, your hands will be as smooth and soft as butter.

2. Wash with warm water, never hot. Hot water tends to strip your skin of its natural oils. Warm water doesn't tend to do this as much.

3. When appropriate, try to use hand sanitizer instead of soap and water. Soap and water strip your skin of essential oils and are more drying to your skin than hand sanitizer (even though there's usually some alcohol in these). If you have a job where you have to wash your hands several times a day (such as a doctor or nurse), then using a hand sanitizer when possible can help prevent your hands from drying out.

Beauty Secret

You don't have to spend a lot of money on hand moisturizers. In fact, you shouldn't. Good facial moisturizers are quite a bit more expensive than good hand moisturizers, so spend your money on your face and save it on your hands. You will spend more on hand moisturizer than on an all-over body moisturizer, however. A good hand moisturizer should withstand several hand washings, whereas body moisturizers aren't typically formulated that way.

If you'd like to make a nice moisturizing hand treatment at home, try this one:

DIY Oats and Moisturizer Hand Treatment

3 heaping tablespoons dry oats (like old-fashioned rolled oats you would use to make oatmeal)

¼ cup water

1 teaspoon baking soda

2 tablespoons sea salt

1. Mix the oats with water in a small blender, like a Magic Bullet, until pureed. Pour the mixture into a small bowl, then add the baking soda and sea salt. Mix together with a spoon or fork.

2. Rub the mixture onto your hands for several minutes to exfoliate them. It will help to remove the upper layer of dead, dry skin cells.

3. Wash the mixture away gently with warm water.

4. Use a powerful, moisturizing barrier cream like Burt's Bees Almond Milk Beeswax Hand Crème, then apply gloves over your hands overnight. Shea butter and beeswax are two of the most powerful moisturizing ingredients in creams today.

5. When you wake up in the morning your hands will be soft and smooth and have fewer wrinkles and less crepey skin.

Beauty Secret

Your hands are looking good—but what about your elbows? For an easy homemade elbow treatment, use the fleshy side of papaya skin to rub on your elbows. Allow the pulp to dry for about twenty minutes, then wash it off and apply moisturizer. Papaya skin is rich in vitamin A and papain, which helps exfoliate dead skin cells. Plus, it's a good excuse to eat more of this antioxidant-rich fruit!

Foot Rejuvenation

Finally, let's not forget those hardworking feet. Our feet get a daily pounding and are probably the most neglected parts of our bodies. Men, especially, take horrible care of their feet, and I've heard many women lamenting that the men in their lives don't get pedicures. If I were to survey women readers about how many of their men have nasty, cracked, disgusting feet, I bet at least 75 percent of them would raise their hands.

I say feet are neglected, but many women take good care of their feet. They get regular pedicures and are great with moisturizing, filing, and keeping them looking great. Not every woman is so diligent about her feet, however. Life gets busy, and if you never look down, then you might forget. If you need a little help in the foot department, then I have a few suggestions:

* **Silk'n Pedi:** The same company that makes my favorite at-home laser hair removal device also makes a nifty, inexpensive little device that can rejuvenate your feet. This handheld, battery-operated device uses exfoliating rollers to smooth away calluses and dead, dry skin, preparing your skin for a great moisturizing cream. For those of you (like my wife) who are a bit grossed out at the thought of getting a pedicure using the same files used on twenty people's feet before you, the Silk'n Pedi may be a great option for you. It can be purchased online for only $29 and is an ✳ AGE FIX FAVORITE.

* **Heel Rescue Superior Moisturizing Foot Cream:** This is a non-greasy, extremely moisturizing cream for the feet. It's best applied before bed, after using the Silk'n Pedi; then put socks on over it to help seal in the moisture. It costs about $12.

* **Denture cleaner:** While you're at it, what about lightening your yellowed toenails? Toenails can get yellow with frequent polish use or because of age and abuse. (If your toenail turns other weird colors, see your doctor or a podiatrist—you could have a fungal infection under there!) To whiten your toenails, just drop a denture-cleaning tablet into a wide bowl or bucket of warm water. While the tablet is dissolving, dip your feet into it. Let your feet soak for ten minutes, then take a washcloth or, even better, a dishwashing sponge, and clean and scrub your feet and toenails.

* **Avocado peel:** This is a very practical way to use the avocado peel that you would normally throw in the garbage. This treatment works so well because the pulp remaining inside the avocado shell is full of skin moisturizers, like those omega-3 fatty acids that are so good for you to eat. The shape of the peel just fits a heel, and the shell itself exfoliates your skin to help remove the top layer of dead, dry, and damaged skin cells. Finally, avocados are full of antioxidants, which are great for fighting off skin-aging free radicals. Here's what to do:

1. After you've cut an avocado in half and scooped out the pit and fruit for your salad or whatever you used it on (and remember, eating avocado provides you with excellent-quality fatty acids that will help keep your skin looking younger!), rub the inside of the scooped peel against your heels for several minutes. The shape of the peel will conform perfectly to your heel.

2. Allow the leftover pulp that sticks on your heels to dry for about ten to fifteen minutes.

3. Wash it off with warm (but not hot) water. (Remember, hot water can dry out your skin.)

4. Finally, apply a good moisturizer afterward, or use extra-virgin olive oil if you want to keep it in the kitchen.

5. To maximize the benefits, do this before bed and apply a sock over the whole thing, then wear the socks overnight to lock in the moisture. Wash it off in the morning during your shower.

Tweaking, fixing, and improving those little annoying parts of your body that bother you really can become a sort of art form, and I hope you will embrace it as fun and affirming rather than disliking yourself for having a few puffy leg veins or being a little sweaty or having scaly feet. Love your body and take care of it, and many of these problems will resolve, so you can stop worrying about them and get back to the business of living your happy life.

10 | AGING GRACEFULLY

Now that you have the tools to keep yourself looking (and feeling) younger, fresher, firmer, and more like *you*, let's talk about what happens next. I can't stop you from aging, but I will give you a final checklist of what to do every day, week, and month for the rest of your life to maintain the work we've done in this book. Learn it, live it, make it part of your routine, and don't be surprised if, as the years roll by, people stare at you and ask, "Why is it that you never age?" or even, "Have you had work done?" Of course, you can answer however you like, but perhaps you will just smile mysteriously. Or tell them that you have a very good doctor. I've organized this by decade, but even if you are somewhere in the middle, read all the decades, because sometimes I want you to keep doing something you've been doing (or could have been doing) from the decade before.

IN YOUR TWENTIES

In your twenties, the main thing to be concerned about is maintaining. You have the benefit of youth, but the goal for the rest of your life is to keep things looking and feeling young. Give up any bad habits that you might have begun during your late teens, such as smoking and eating foods that are bad for you, like fast foods and processed foods. The goal is to establish a healthy lifestyle that you will maintain for a long, long time. You can also:

Prepare: Use a **cleanser appropriate for your skin type** (check out chapter 4 if you aren't sure what that might be).

Treat: Your skin should look great, since you are young. Therefore, you don't need to spend a lot of money on prescription-strength products (many people in their twenties can't afford them anyway).

* Begin applying an inexpensive, over-the-counter **antioxidant cream** in the morning. **Vitamin C creams** are plentiful and are great for your skin in your twenties.

* If you are able, you can also purchase an inexpensive **retinol cream**. Unless you have acne issues, prescription-strength tretinoin is probably more aggressive than you need, so retinol will do. It starts fighting off the aging process at this stage in your life. It also helps the cellular turnover of your skin and can very gradually lighten any early sun spots.

Protect: *Sunblock is the key* during your twenties. Although a golden tan might be considered attractive, any sun damage your skin gets in your twenties will begin to show up as aging in the next ten to twenty years. You can do a lot to prevent that now. Think ahead! Apply sunblock every morning as a part of your daily moisturizer or separately.

Interventions: Don't waste your money on invasive or expensive treatments in your twenties. This is the time to enjoy your youthful face and body!

IN YOUR THIRTIES

In your thirties, the main thing to be concerned about is early aging. If you aren't taking good care of yourself, you will begin to see age-related changes during this time. Many people look great in their twenties, no matter the lifestyle they lead. Youth allows the body to bounce back without much difficulty. Sorry to say that begins changing in your thirties. If you haven't done so, now is the time to start leading a healthy lifestyle. Cut back on sugar, processed food, and unhealthy fats, and focus on eating foods rich in antioxidants, omega-3 fatty acids, and whole grains. Your thirties are also the time when treating age-related changes becomes just as important as preventing aging.

Prepare: Continue to use a **cleanser suited for your skin type**. This is also a time to begin **exfoliating** your skin a couple of times a week if you aren't already. Your skin cell turnover slows down in your thirties, so you can really benefit from this now.

Treat: Now is also the time to consider more aggressive antiaging treatments for your skin.

* If you haven't started a **retinol cream**, your thirties is a great time to start. Better yet, if your skin tolerates it, see a plastic surgeon or dermatologist for **prescription-strength tretinoin**. This can be your number one antiaging cream for the rest of your life.

✳ Also continue with your **antioxidant cream**, such as **vitamin C.** If you have the financial means, then consider a higher-end version, as these formulations may be more stable and effective.

✳ Begin using an **eye cream**, preferably one that contains **retinol with rich moisturizers**. Most people start noticing changes in the thin skin of the eyelids in their thirties, so this is a good time to get started treating them separately from the rest of your face. See chapter 7 for suggestions.

Protect: Moisturizer, then sunblock, sunblock, sunblock. Oh, and did I mention sunblock?

Interventions: Your thirties are the decade to start thinking about minor treatments to keep your skin and body looking youthful.

✳ **No-downtime lasers and peels** are great ways to exfoliate your skin and keep it looking smooth, tight, and youthful. More aggressive lasers and peels probably aren't needed at this stage, unless you are treating a specific condition.

✳ Many people begin injections of **Botox** now to smooth newly developing crow's-feet and frown lines. These easy treatments will help to prevent these wrinkles from becoming settled and getting too deep.

✳ Many women also begin noninvasive **cellulite treatments** in their thirties. You're still young enough to rock a two-piece, but a little help with your skin can make you look practically indistinguishable from those twenty-year-olds!

IN YOUR FORTIES

In your forties, you have probably noticed additional and more obvious wrinkling and other visible signs of aging. The life you've led up to this point will show in your forties, and your youthful indiscretions will catch up with you. People who've led an unhealthy lifestyle will look older than people who've been practicing healthy habits since their twenties. But that doesn't mean you can't still have fun—if you haven't already discovered their charms, now is a good time to learn about the benefits of dark chocolate and red wine. Become a connoisseur of these healthy, antioxidant-rich foods (making sure to partake in them conservatively). Our forties is also the time when the face visibly loses volume or gets more gaunt. This is therefore the decade when most men and women consider more invasive and expensive treatments to look younger.

Prepare: Cleanse. Also continue exfoliating several times a week, as your skin is definitely turning over at a slower pace in your forties. If you haven't yet, consider buying a **Clarisonic-type device.**

Treat: Stay the course, with a few additions when relevant:

* Continue **retinol or tretinoin** as your main antiaging cream.

* Continue an **antioxidant cream,** such as **vitamin C.**

* Also continue with a good **eye cream.**

* This is also a good time to consider adding a regular **skin-brightening cream,** such as one with **niacinamide** or **kojic acid.** You may notice your skin developing age spots more quickly and easily than ever before.

* If your age spots are significant, then see a plastic surgeon or dermatologist to start a regimen of prescription-strength **hydroquinone.** Once the spots have disappeared, return to your usual regimen of a nonprescription skin brightener, as you shouldn't be on hydroquinone indefinitely.

Protect: Moisturizer. And I hate to belabor the point, but…sunblock.

Interventions: The interventions from your thirties still apply, with a few additions:

* **Regular no-downtime chemical peels or laser treatments** can continue to rejuvenate the collagen in your skin.

* You may also consider a more aggressive skin-tightening and rejuvenating treatment, such as a series of **moderate-depth chemical peels or fractional laser treatments,** if you want to see a more dramatic change.

* **Botox** can keep your forehead, frown lines, and crow's-feet areas as smooth as they were in your twenties.

* Consider **fillers for nasolabial folds and facial revolumizing.** The nasolabial folds (deep grooves extending between the sides of your nose and corners of your mouth) become more prominent in most people in their forties. Injectable fillers like **Restylane** and **Juvederm** are great treatments for this. You may also notice that your cheeks are becoming more hollow and your lips thinner. **Voluma** and **Sculptra** are nice, nonsurgical options for subtle volumizing of the cheeks, and a conservative amount of Restylane or Juvederm can be used to plump the lips back to what they used to be.

* **Cellulite treatments** are popular at this age. Yes, even in your forties you can rock that two-piece! Noninvasive cellulite treatments, especially ones that can take inches off (see chapter 8), can be a great way to help keep your figure.

IN YOUR FIFTIES

For women, menopause probably causes more aging effects than anything else, and most women go through menopause in their late forties or early fifties. As hormonal changes ramp up, women often notice their skin getting thinner and drier, so you may benefit from topical products that are more moisturizing. In virtually everyone, women and men, our skin begins to droop visibly in our fifties, in addition to the changes that we noticed in our forties (fine lines, age spots, and cellulite). Depressing, right? Wrong! There are many things that you can do in your fifties to continue looking young and vibrant. Some of these, unfortunately, may be invasive and include some downtime. But in today's world, I truly believe that fifty is the new thirty. Celebrities like Michelle Pfeiffer, Tom Cruise, and Vanessa Williams have proven this!

Prepare: Cleanse. You may benefit from switching to a **creamier cleanser** that retains more of your skin's essential oils. Keep **exfoliating**, too. Your skin needs this now more than ever, as the normal cellular mechanisms for skin cell turnover have definitely slowed down.

Treat: It's time to make a few more tweaks to your skin treatments:

* The thinner and drier skin that accompanies menopause may be more sensitive to the drying effects of regular tretinoin. If this is the case, you may want to switch to the **moisturizing, emollient form of tretinoin, called Renova or ReFissa**.

* If prescription-strength tretinoin (in any form) is too aggressive and drying, then consider **retinol creams,** or substitute these with a serum or cream that contains **growth hormone or peptides**. Even if you are tolerating your tretinoin or retinol, adding growth factor and/or peptide creams can provide even more of an age-reducing effect!

* Continue with a **skin-brightening cream (non-hydroquinone)** to fight off age spots and keep your skin looking luminous.

* Continue with an **antioxidant cream**.

* Continue with an **eye cream**—if you notice that your lower eyelids are getting puffy, one with **caffeine** can help reduce this.

* Use prescription-strength **hydroquinone** as needed for short periods of time (as directed by your plastic surgeon or dermatologist) to reduce sun and age spots.

Protect: In addition to your old standbys, **moisturizer** and **sunblock**, add a **night cream**, preferably one that contains antiaging ingredients such as **retinol, growth factors, or peptides**. Menopause can rob your skin of the moisture it used to have, so a rich, moisturizing night cream can be very helpful in rejuvenating your skin while you sleep.

Interventions: This is the decade when you may begin to consider interventions you hadn't considered before:

* Use **regular no-downtime chemical peels or laser treatments** for maintenance, and consider being a little more intensive with **moderate-depth chemical peels or more aggressive laser treatments** to tighten skin and improve fine lines.

* **Botox and fillers** can continue to make a big difference in your fifties.

* You can't prevent a certain degree of sagging, but skin-tightening **cellulite treatments** can still help your figure to look at least a decade younger.

* The fifties are when some people begin to consider **surgical options**, as issues such as drooping eyelids or neck become more noticeable and annoying. Most women, however, are happy to simply ramp up their regular beauty routine and keep exercising for the youngest possible look without surgery.

IN YOUR SIXTIES, SEVENTIES, AND BEYOND

The changes that you begin to see in your fifties (such as sagging skin, deeper wrinkles, and dryness) unfortunately progress in your sixties and seventies and throughout the rest of your golden years. There's no way to prevent this from occurring, but all of the recommendations of how to treat your skin in your fifties should slow this process down significantly. Continue with these recommendations, and you'll be doing everything you can to keep aging at bay. If you need more inspiration, think of the many celebs who look fantastic in their sixties, like Christie Brinkley, Denzel Washington, and Jane Seymour. Your sixties are the time when surgery can often provide the most dramatic results. Although surgery isn't for everyone, this is the time most people make their definitive decision on actual surgery. Either it's not for them, or they want to obtain the dramatic changes in their appearance that can accompany it. Do what you feel is right for you.

Once you get into the habit of caring for and maintaining your skin and your body, you will realize that you have this youth-and-beauty thing *down*. Sure, we all age. None of us can look like twenty-two-year-olds forever (and would you really *want* to?). But every single one of us can look pretty darn good for our age. It's all just a matter of taking good care, and taking advantage of science and technology, as well as the products of the natural world when they are available to you.

A FINAL WORD

In this book we've covered many ways to look younger and change your figure to more closely resemble the one you always wanted, but in the end, I hope you will always remember that it's really not all that important how you look. What really matters is how you feel about yourself. Surveys reveal that confidence is the feature most attractive to most people, and although we all have our own perceived flaws and our own insecurities (even supermodels and the most glamorous Hollywood actors and actresses), the best thing you can do for yourself and your life is to be happy with who you are right here, right now. I meet so many people who are so concerned about their appearance (and tiny perceived flaws) that they allow it to run or ruin their lives. Don't let that happen to you. Don't let others make you feel unattractive. Don't let anyone convince you to have anything done that you don't want to have done. No one truly needs cosmetic surgery.

If there is one thing that I've learned in the past sixteen years as a plastic surgeon, it's that being healthy is the key to retaining our youth. In the end, that's really what the Age Fix is all about. Following the Age-Fix healthy diet guidelines, exercising regularly, taking care of your skin, smelling the proverbial flowers every so often, and having a positive outlook on life are truly the best ways to stay young forever. If you take no other advice from me, I hope you will take this to heart.

And if you still want to change something? If you still want to look younger, just because you enjoy feeling good and looking good, just because you want to do it for yourself? Then by all means, try the tips, strategies, and suggestions in this book. Nobody will do everything I recommend, nor should they, but find the suggestions that speak to you—and most of all, have fun taking care of yourself. It's your body and your life, and taking care of yourself will make you feel better every day, no matter how many years young you happen to be.

BONUS CHAPTER

The Age Fix Update by Anthony Youn, MD

The fields of beauty and plastic surgery are constantly changing. It seems that every week there is a new device that is FDA-cleared, a new cream touted as "better than Botox," or a new beauty trend to consider. If it's hard for doctors to keep up with all the new treatments, procedures, and products, then I can't imagine how difficult it is for the patient or consumer! Although *The Age Fix* contains the most up-to-date information on beauty and antiaging of any book currently available, more than a year has passed since the book was first published.

There have been many changes in the fields of beauty and plastic surgery that I'm sure you'd love to know about. In this chapter, I'll describe to you a number of new, revolutionary, and fascinating treatments being performed this very minute in select plastic surgeons' and dermatologists' offices. I'll share with you several new or heretofore unpublicized antiaging products to consider trying. I'll even give you a handful of new DIY recipes to try at home to make your skin look and feel younger.

YOUR FACE

Kybella

Have you heard of **Kybella** yet? This is the most exciting new treatment to hit my office in quite some time. Kybella was FDA-approved in April 2015 and is a great new injectable treatment to get rid of a double chin. Our office has been packed with patients asking about and receiving this treatment, so I thought it would be a good place to start.

Kybella is composed of deoxycholic acid, a naturally occurring molecule in the body that aids in the breakdown and absorption of dietary fat. When injected into the subcutaneous fat under the chin (the layer of fat below the skin), it can cause the fat to dissolve and the body to dispose of it by natural processes. It's like magic! There is one caveat, though: Kybella doesn't tighten or lift the skin. The best results occur in people who have good skin tone but want to get rid of some extra fat.

The actual procedure is really quick and can be nearly painless. A doctor starts by marking the area, with care taken to avoid injecting close to nerves or the organs of the neck. At this time, I prefer to inject a local anesthetic to numb the area, though some doctors just use ice for pain control. The Kybella is then injected into the fat under the chin, taking about three to four minutes for the actual treatment.

Most patients experience quite intense burning for about ten minutes after the injections, although with the local anesthetic they usually don't feel a thing. Within a couple of hours, swelling sets in, sometimes accompanied by a temporary numbness. These symptoms typically resolve within a couple of weeks, and most of my patients notice a nice change in just one or two treatments, although two to four treatments are usually required for maximal results.

The best candidates for Kybella are between the ages of about eighteen and fifty. For many people over the age of fifty, loose skin can become an issue, especially since Kybella doesn't actively tighten the skin. Because of this, some doctors have been combining Kybella with nonsurgical skin-tightening treatments, like **Ultherapy**. The jury is still out on how effective these modalities are when combined.

The main problem I have with Kybella is the price. Each Kybella treatment costs patients between $1,000 and $2,000. With the average patient needing two to four treatments, this can really add up. That's why I encourage anyone thinking about Kybella to consider liposuction as well. Liposuction under the chin is what I consider a "weekend neck lift." It can be performed with minimal pain and downtime, low cost, and tiny scars. However, it's still surgery and can cost upward of $2,000 to $4,000. Make sure to discuss both of these treatments with your plastic surgeon before deciding on which one is right for you.

One final question that people ask me is whether Kybella can be used to reduce fat on other parts of the body. Currently, it's approved only for use below the chin, but I've heard some doctors are using it for other parts of the body, too. Keep in mind that this is considered an "off-label" use and may be riskier than just injecting it into a double chin.

CoolMini

What if you want to get rid of your double chin, but you don't want to be poked with needles? Now you have the option of freezing the fat with the **CoolMini** applicator from **CoolSculpting**. I talk about CoolSculpting in chapter 8, but to summarize, it's a device that freezes the fat of the abdomen, hips, and thighs, causing it to be irreversibly damaged. The body then clears this damaged fat over the span of several weeks. Studies have shown an average fat reduction of around 25 percent after just one treatment. Unfortunately, the CoolSculpting applicator is too large to use for the small, delicate area under the chin.

In September 2015, the FDA cleared the CoolMini applicator, which can be used to freeze the fat under the chin. Studies have shown an average reduction of 20 percent of the thickness of the fat after a single treatment or two treatments spaced six weeks apart. The most dramatic results occur one to two months after the treatment. Each treatment costs approximately $750 to $1,000.

So, which should you choose to get rid of your double chin? Liposuction, Kybella, or CoolMini?

If you want a quick and dramatic improvement, are not opposed to a tiny scar under your chin, and want to know exactly how much you will spend up front, then consider liposuction first. Recovery time is usually a weekend, but bruising and swelling can take much longer to resolve. In the end, though, the results are consistently impressive.

If you don't want surgery, aren't afraid of needles, and want a dramatic change, then Kybella may be your best choice. Kybella can reduce your fat just as impressively as liposuction, albeit with more treatments and subsequently more cost. In general, you begin to approach the cost of surgery after about two treatments with Kybella. The benefits of Kybella, though, are no scars, no surgery, and no downtime.

Finally, if you are OK with a more subtle change and don't want surgery or injections, then CoolMini could be a good option for you. It's the least expensive and invasive of the three choices but may have less dramatic results.

Skyn Iceland Face-Lift-in-a-Bag

Speaking of cool, one of the newest and most popular beauty treatments is adherent gel strips that produce a refreshing, chilling sensation to the skin. These are often used on the eyelids in place of the tried-and-true cold slices of cucumber. **Skyn Iceland** produces gel strips that are infused with a plethora of moisturizers and antioxidants to soothe and hydrate the skin, and even temporarily reduce fine lines. You can buy these gel strips for each specific part of the face (forehead, smile lines, or under the eyes) or as a package called the **Face-Lift-in-a-Bag** ($19.50). After just ten minutes, your skin feels smooth, hydrated, and even relaxed. It's perfect to use after a long day at work.

DIY Lemonade Scrub

Exfoliation is one of the cornerstones of good skin care. Here is a fun little recipe you can make at home to smooth and polish your skin:

2 tablespoons honey
2 tablespoons granulated sugar
1 tablespoon lemon juice

Mix these ingredients together, and then apply the mixture to your face. Gently rub your face with this scrub in circular motions, allowing time for these great ingredients to affect your skin. This scrub combines the moisturizing and soothing properties of honey with the mild exfoliation of sugar granules and lemon juice (containing citric acid, an AHA). Sugar may not be good to ingest, but it can be a great exfoliating agent.

Keep in mind that this one can be a little messy. And try not to drip any of the scrub on the bathroom floor, for the honey will make your toes stick to the tile or carpet.

Rhofade

Rosacea is one of the most frustrating conditions to treat. It's an inflammatory skin condition that affects millions of Americans. If you suffer from rosacea, then you know it involves facial flushing and redness that can be triggered by sun exposure, stress, weather, foods, and exercise. There are a lot of treatments for rosacea, including lasers and creams, but none of them has risen above the others as the gold standard of treatment.

Rhofade is an exciting new prescription topical cream that can reduce the redness of rosacea, literally within minutes. It was FDA-approved in January 2017 and just may be a game changer for people who suffer from this condition. The effects of one topical application can last up to twelve hours, and the science behind the product is strong. It must be obtained via a prescription or at a physician's office, so don't look for it at the department store. As of this writing, I don't have a lot of experience with it, but many dermatologists are bullish on what this revolutionary cream can do for rosacea sufferers.

Restylane Silk, Defyne, and Refyne

Several new injectable fillers have hit the market since the original publication of *The Age Fix.* One new member of the Restylane family is **Restylane Silk.** (If you are outside the United States, it's called Restylane Fine Lines.) This filler is FDA-approved for filling in wrinkles around the mouth (the so-called "smoker's lines"). It's also a nice treatment to plump up the lips, since it's a finer substance that feels a little softer than most other injectable fillers. Restylane Silk lasts about six months on average. The cost is about the same as regular Restylane, ranging from $500 to $750 per syringe.

An interesting new pair of injectable fillers are **Restylane Refyne** and **Restylane Defyne**. These products have been used in Europe since 2010 under the name Emervel, but were approved by the FDA in December 2016 under the names Restylane Refyne and Restylane Defyne. Although they are both hyaluronic acid fillers, they are different from all the other fillers being used today because they're specifically made to be extremely smooth. Normally, the knock on injectable fillers is that they can sometimes make the skin look stiff and unnatural. These two new fillers utilize XpresHAn Technology to create the smoothest results we have seen so far with any filler. For this reason, they are great for injecting around the mouth, lips, and lower face. Restylane Refyne is a thinner substance, so it's used for fine lines. Restylane Defyne is a thicker filler, so it's better for deeper wrinkles. Both of them are shown to last approximately one year. In my practice, these two fillers are fast becoming patient favorites for wrinkles of the lower face.

Juvederm Volbella and Vollure

Juvederm Volbella, a competitor of Restylane Silk, was FDA-approved in May 2016 and hit doctors' offices in October 2016. Volbella is a great option for smoothing the fine lines of the upper and lower lip. Prior to Volbella, all of the injectable hyaluronic acid fillers were too thick to treat fine lines. Instead of filling in wrinkles, they'd often result in ridges and lumps. Volbella is so fine a substance it fills in even some of the thinnest lines without creating these problems. Unfortunately, the characteristic that makes it great for smoothing fine lines also makes it a poor choice for plumping up lips. It's too thin and spreads out too much to do that.

Volbella lasts 6 to 12 months and costs about $500 to $750. If you want to smooth your smoker's lines but don't want fuller lips, then this could be a great treatment for you.

Juvederm Vollure was FDA-approved in March 2017 for the treatment of deep, moderate wrinkles, such as the nasolabial folds. It works similarly to Juvederm Ultra Plus, but lasts much longer, approximately a year and a half. As of this writing, I haven't used it a lot, but if it's anywhere near as good as Juvederm Ultra or Juvederm Voluma, then it just might become the standard for filling and smoothing the nasolabial folds. If you are thinking of having your nasolabial folds treated, ask your doctor about this new and exciting filler.

Bliss Two-Step Lip Enhancing and Rejuvenating System

This is a nice inexpensive system that I shared on *The Rachael Ray Show*. If you have dry, chapped, or thin lips, then this is the treatment for you. Start by using the **Bliss Fabulips Pout-O-Matic Lip-Perfecting System**. Say that five times fast! This small, $48 device combines with the **Fabulips Sugar Lip Scrub** to exfoliate and buff away dry, flaking skin from your lips, leaving them soft and smooth. The head of the device rotates at more than 450 rotations per minute. The sugar crystals gently exfoliate the lips and also taste great. Once your lips are properly exfoliated, apply the **Bliss Fabulips Instant Lip Plumper** ($22). This lip gloss instantly plumps your lips in two ways. It aggressively moisturizes them with squalene and creates a mild irritation / tingling sensation with peppermint oil. This two-step system is perfect to rejuvenate tired, dried-out lips and give you a plump pout again.

DIY Peach-and-Olive-Oil Mask

This is a very simple and easy DIY way to hydrate your skin and infuse it with a healthy combination of antiaging alpha hydroxy acids, free-radical-fighting antioxidants, and moisturizing squalene. Take one half of a peach and peel off the skin. Mash the peach with a fork until it's fairly soft. Then, combine the mashed peach with one tablespoon of olive oil, and mix together. Apply this mixture to your skin, and let it sit for twenty minutes. Then, rinse off with warm water. Your skin will feel smoother and more hydrated afterward.

Face Yoga

Have you heard about this relatively new trend? Many videos on YouTube demonstrate how performing face yoga poses can actually make you look younger. Do I believe it? Not really.

This comes back to the face exercises I talk about in chapter 2. Making various extreme facial expressions can actually contribute to deeper wrinkles instead of smoothing them out. Repetitive facial expressions can cause the underlying muscles to create deeper and deeper grooves in the skin. This is the reason why we develop crow's-feet wrinkles, frown lines, and horizontal forehead wrinkles as we age.

So, is there anything good about doing face yoga? Yes!

One prominent part of face yoga involves relaxing your face. Relaxing and training your muscles of facial expression *not* to contract is a great way to keep wrinkles at bay. It's like a natural form of Botox! So, if you're thinking about doing face yoga to look younger, I recommend that you skip making the extreme facial expressions and instead focus on its relaxation techniques. Those can provide a (small) help in looking younger.

Microneedling with and without Growth Factors

One of the hottest treatments in my practice right now is **Microneedling**. I briefly mention this treatment in chapter 9 as a new option for acne scarring, but over the past year or so, it has exploded in popularity as technological advances have expanded its cosmetic indications. Microneedling is now one of the premier skin rejuvenation treatments in med spas and doctors' offices throughout the United States.

You may have seen handheld rollers with tiny needles that, when rolled on the skin, cause microtrauma to it. These "dermal rollers" make tiny punctures in the skin, typically less than one millimeter deep, causing the skin to be temporarily damaged. When the skin is damaged, the healing process causes the collagen in the skin to heal in a tighter, smoother fashion. This is also how lasers and chemical peels cause our skin to look more youthful.

The problem with the handheld dermal rollers is that the round shape of the roller can cause the depth of the punctures to vary. Therefore, several companies now manufacture handheld automated microneedling devices. These devices can be calibrated to create a very consistent depth of micropuncture, from one to two millimeters or even deeper. This allows the doctor or aesthetician to tailor the treatment to how aggressive the patient wants it. The deeper the punctures, the more trauma to the skin and the greater the changes.

Microneedling is now being combined with the topical application of growth factors for an even greater rejuvenating effect to the skin. The idea is that the tiny punctures created by microneedling can act as channels into the deeper skin (the dermis). Applying a growth factor serum immediately after the microneedling treatment allows it to penetrate deep into the skin to rejuvenate it. Many practices have seen great changes to the skin by using this potent microneedling and growth-factor combination. The skin becomes smoother and tighter and has fewer fine lines.

Some doctors are combining microneedling with the application of **platelet-rich plasma (PRP)**. In this process, the doctor or nurse draws the patient's blood, spins it down, removes the platelets, and applies this substance (PRP) on the treated skin. The PRP is chock-full of a patient's own all-natural growth factors. Combining microneedling with PRP can look pretty gruesome, but many doctors swear by it. In my practice, we're combining microneedling with **Tensage Growth Factor Serum**. My aestheticians (who perform the microneedling for my patients) don't want to deal with vials of blood, so we prefer the much cleaner, commercially available Tensage.

These automated microneedling treatments can take about forty-five minutes in a doctor's office or medical spa and can range from $200 for a superficial treatment to almost $1,000 when PRP is used. Downtime is typically a day or two, unless you have a deeper treatment. It's very important to inform the doctor or aesthetician if you have a history of cold sores so that he or she can prescribe you an antiviral medication to prevent an eruption after the procedure.

YOUR EYES

XAF5 Ointment

What do you think about an ointment applied to the bags under the eyes that shrinks fat cells and reduces puffiness? Well, I have recently heard about a new topical treatment that might be able to do just that and make a huge impact in the field of plastic surgery. Early results reportedly show that an experimental ointment from Topokine Therapeutics called **XAF5** can create a nice improvement in the puffiness under the eyes after just five weeks of topical application. The proprietary active ingredient is currently being tested by the FDA. There is no set timetable for its release, but I'll be monitoring this one closely. A topical product has never been proven to melt underlying fat, so this one could be a true game changer. I'll post any updates on the XAF5 Ointment on my free monthly e-newsletter, so feel free to sign up on my website, www.dryoun.com, for the latest on this exciting treatment.

Garnier Clearly Brighter Anti-Dark-Circle Roller

In the meantime, are there any effective, noninvasive options to improve dark circles under the eyes? In chapter 7, I mention some quick-fix products that act as a "shrink-wrap" to reduce puffiness of the lower eyelids. In addition to these products, I have a few new options to consider.

Garnier sells a nifty, inexpensive treatment that can immediately improve the appearance of dark circles under the eyes. The **Clearly Brighter Anti-Dark-Circle Roller** is a two-in-one product that combines a mild concealer with a number of skin-care ingredients to make a very nice improvement to the under-eye area. In addition to the makeup component, it contains the moisturizers dimethicone and squalene to fill in fine lines and caffeine to tighten the skin. The product is very easy to apply and costs only about $12.99. With some minor blending using the pad of your pinkie or ring finger, you can get a really nice, natural improvement in the appearance under the eyes. I use it for my under-eye puffiness before TV tapings when we don't have a professional makeup artist on hand.

RoC Retinol Correxion Eye Cream

The Garnier product above is great to hide under-eye puffiness temporarily. But if you truly want to reverse the aging of the under-eye skin, I strongly encourage you to consider using a retinol-based cream. The **RoC Retinol Correxion Eye Cream** is a silky, hydrating eye cream that combines moisturizing glycerin with antiaging retinol. Apply it to the sensitive under-eye skin using your pinkie or ring finger every morning and evening. For an eyelid cream, it's very affordable, too, costing only $22.99—perhaps less if you search around online. You can't get a much better lower-eyelid cream for the price.

YOUR BREASTS

The field of breast enhancement has seen some interesting developments recently, too. Let's start by talking about vacation breasts.

Vacation Breasts

One doctor in New York City has recently begun advertising instant breast enhancement, or "vacation breasts," as nicknamed by the media. In this procedure, the doctor injects a large amount of saline (saltwater) into the breasts as a way to enlarge them temporarily. Within a day or two, the body reabsorbs the saline, and the breasts return to their normal size—all for $2,500.

It's an invasive procedure, and although it doesn't involve cutting, it does involve long needles and, I would assume, a good deal of pain. Some patients who've been interviewed for the news segments on vacation breasts claim that it's a useful way for them to "test-drive" implants.

That's a very expensive test-drive!

So, what can go wrong? Well, if the doctor is very careful, the risks are probably minimal because it's only salt water that is injected. However, if the doctor injects too deeply, then he or she could theoretically collapse a lung. This isn't a procedure that I perform or recommend to my patients. If you really want to test-drive implants, try the **Rice Test**. This is a very simple way to try out various breast implant sizes in the privacy of your own home. All you do is take a calf-high nylon stocking, fill it with a measured amount of rice (the average implant volume in my practice is 350 ml), flatten the rice into a disc shape, and stuff it into the front of your non-padded bra. Add or subtract rice 25 ml at a time until you see the size you like. Of note, silicone-gel breast implants usually come in 25 ml increments (i.e. 300 ml, 325 ml, 350 ml, etc.), so stick with 25 ml increments to be most accurate. I recently demonstrated how to do this on *The Rachael Ray Show*, and you can see the video on my website at www.dryoun.com/plastic-surgery/services/breast/breast-augmentation.

OK, now that I've discussed preparing for a breast augmentation, let's dive into the actual surgery. There are two new breast implants that every woman considering this operation must be aware of. Let's start with the newest silicone gel implant.

Natrelle Inspira Breast Implants

Fifteen years ago, we had basically one type of breast implant available for use in the United States: the traditional saline implant. Today, we have a plethora of options. The new **Natrelle Inspira** family of implants is a modification of the silicone gel-filled breast implants commonly used today. There are two main differences. The first is that the Natrelle Inspira has a higher silicone-gel-fill ratio. This means that the Inspira has more silicone gel packed into the implant shell than do other similar implants, making it look rounder and causing fewer wrinkles and ripples. The second is that the actual silicone filling these implants is more cohesive, or solid, than the silicone gel that is otherwise used today. This allows the implant to keep its shape, similar to the "gummy bear" implants I wrote about earlier. These implants can be especially helpful for women who already have breast implants and have issues with them rippling or wrinkling.

The Natrelle Inspira comes in three different levels of firmness or cohesion. There is the softer Natrelle Inspira, the moderately firm Natrelle Inspira Soft Touch, and the firm Natrelle Inspira Cohesive. The firmer and more cohesive the implant, the less wrinkling and rippling, but the more it retains its round shape, causing the entire breast to look rounder.

Breasts come in all shapes and sizes. It's great that we now have such a wide variety of silicone gel implants to accommodate everyone's individual anatomy.

The Ideal Implant

Yes, I know, I know. We already discussed the **Ideal Implant** in chapter 8, but now I have a lot more information on it that I'd like to share with you.

The Ideal Implant is the newest saline-filled breast implant on the market. It contains internal chambers that allow the liquid inside to move around more smoothly compared with a traditional saline implant. This makes the implant (and therefore the breast) look and feel more natural than a traditional saline implant, with less wrinkling and rippling. Some patients find that the results approach the natural look and feel of a silicone-gel implant.

Another added benefit that most doctors and patients aren't aware of is that if this implant breaks, which happens very rarely, only one internal chamber deflates. This allows the patient more time to get the implant switched out before the pocket shrinks. Typically, when a traditional saline implant breaks, the implant completely deflates like a balloon. This causes the pocket it's in to shrink as well. Waiting too long to get the implant switched out can make it necessary for the plastic surgeon to reopen the pocket. This can become an extensive, bloody operation. Because the Ideal Implant has two inner shells, if one breaks, the implant remains partially inflated, allowing the patient more time to switch out the implant. This can mean the difference between a simple implant-exchange operation, which could take fifteen minutes, and an operation to reopen the entire breast implant pocket, which could take an hour and a half.

The major negative of the Ideal Implant is its price. Because Ideal Implant Inc. is still a small company (and, as of this writing, only a few hundred plastic surgeons around the country have access to the Ideal Implant), the cost of the Ideal Implant is about twice that of a traditional saline implant. However, I predict that the Ideal Implant will eventually make the traditional saline implant obsolete.

Thoroughly confused as to which implant to choose? Before making your decision about which breast implants may be right for you, it's extremely important that you read the next section.

BREAST IMPLANT-ASSOCIATED ANAPLASTIC LARGE CELL LYMPHOMA (BIA-ALCL)

A very concerning type of cancer has been discovered that appears to be related to having breast implants. Anaplastic Large Cell Lymphoma (ALCL) is a type of malignant cancer that arises in the scar tissue (capsule) surrounding a breast implant. It most commonly presents as a spontaneous fluid collection approximately eight to ten years after the original surgery. It can also present as a breast mass or as swollen lymph nodes.

As of this writing, there have been 359 reported cases to the FDA and 126 confirmed cases reported to the official database. All of the patients who have had confirmed BIA-ALCL have a history of a textured-surface breast implant. There have been no confirmed cases of BIA-ALCL in women who've had only smooth implants. BIA-ALCL doesn't appear related to the implant fill or type of surgery; both silicone and saline implants, cosmetic and reconstructive, have reported cases of this rare form of cancer. There appears to be a geographic or genetic influence to BIA-ALCL, however, with many cases reported in Australia but very few in Asia.

So if you have breast implants, what should you do?

First, do not panic. This is a very rare disease. There are millions of women with breast implants, and although I do believe the cases of BIA-ALCL are underreported, it's still extremely unlikely that it will happen to you. However, it's very important that you are informed and proactive. Find out whether you have textured breast implants, and pay special attention if you do. Get your regular medical exams and mammograms. See your plastic surgeon immediately if you notice changes in your breast shape or enlarged lymph nodes.

What if you are considering breast implants? Breast implants are still considered safe, effective, and the gold standard for enhancing the breasts. If you and your plastic surgeon are considering textured implants, then I encourage you to discuss the link between BIA-ALCL and textured implants to determine whether using a textured implant is still the best option for you. Many plastic surgeons continue to use these types of implants with great results.

For more information on BIA-ALCL, please visit the American Society of Plastic Surgeons web page dedicated to this topic: www.plasticsurgery.org/alcl.

YOUR BODY

SculpSure

In chapter 8, I describe numerous devices that are currently used to reduce fat noninvasively. These include **CoolSculpting**, **Vanquish**, **UltraShape**, and many more. Each of these options causes irreversible damage to fat pockets in a different way: by freezing them, heating them with ultrasound, blasting them with radiofrequency, and even modifying them with cold lasers.

SculpSure is the newest entry into this crowded field of noninvasive fat reducers. It's made by Cynosure, the same company that developed Smartlipo, and is the first heat-based laser that is FDA-cleared for noninvasive reduction of fat in the abdomen and flanks. Some doctors are also using it on other parts of the body. Each treatment takes about twenty-five minutes (less than the one hour of CoolSculpting), and typically only one treatment is necessary to start seeing results.

Studies have shown that one treatment of SculpSure can reduce the thickness of fat by an average of 24 percent, similar to the results described for CoolSculpting.[37] As with the other noninvasive fat reducers, results can take six weeks to be visible, with up to twelve weeks for maximal reduction. We recently acquired SculpSure in my office and are finding that patients get the best results after two treatments, each spaced about six weeks apart.

The great thing about SculpSure is that you can treat up to four areas at once! It has four treatment heads, each about the size of a deck of cards. These four heads can be lined up next to each other for treating one large area (like the abdomen) or separated to treat multiple areas (off-label like the arms and flanks). There is some temporary discomfort involved, but the recovery appears to be much easier than CoolSculpting.

SculpSure has offered my patients another good option to achieve what I consider the Holy Grail of plastic surgery: fat loss without dieting, exercise, or surgery. And that's a big deal for us!

ZO Skin Health Oraser Body Emulsion Plus

The vast majority of moisturizers for our hands and body do only that: moisturize. **Oraser Body Emulsion Plus** is a nongreasy body moisturizer from ZO Skin Health. It is one of the few moisturizers that also actively reverse the aging of our skin. It does this via a combination of retinol (in just the right concentration so as not to irritate the skin), exfoliating papain extract, and antioxidants. It feels silky smooth and is absorbed quickly. Although at $95 it's a splurge, it is one product I use on my skin every day. For best results, apply this body moisturizer to your skin within three minutes of showering to lock in the moisture. This is especially important to keep your skin hydrated during the cold, dry winter months in northern climates. Very highly recommended!

Aveeno Skin Relief 24-hr Moisturizing Lotion

Although this body moisturizer won't make your skin any younger, it's a very inexpensive way ($10 for a large eighteen-ounce bottle) to moisturize your skin. It provides lasting relief, unlike some moisturizers that seem to wear off after just a couple of hours. It also won't make your skin feel oily or greasy. I highly recommend it for use in dry climates or during a cold winter. Your skin will thank you for it.

Cellfina

There is no permanent cure for cellulite—or is there?

Cellfina is a new, FDA-cleared, minimally invasive treatment for the long-term reduction of cellulite. It reduces cellulite in a completely different way from any of the treatments described in this book. If you recall, one of the main causes of cellulite dimpling is the thick, fibrous bands that connect the muscle fascia to the overlying skin. Cellfina is a small device that uses a specialized needle to cut these bands, releasing them and causing the dimpling to improve. Although Cellfina is an invasive procedure, it's not surgery.

Studies show the results with Cellfina can be seen in as little as three days and can last two years, possibly more. Best of all, patient satisfaction at two years was a whopping 96 percent. The procedure takes about forty-five minutes but does have some pain associated with it, necessitating a local anesthetic.

There's still no cure for cellulite, but Cellfina appears to be very effective for small areas of dimpling. It's definitely an exciting new treatment for women (and men) who want to improve their cellulite.

St. Ives Smoothing Apricot Exfoliating Body Wash

I've always been a sucker for beauty products that smell like apricots; I think the scent is fresh and clean. Therefore, this exfoliating body wash by St. Ives is one of my favorites. It contains tiny pumice crystals (not the beads that the government wisely banned) that exfoliate the upper layer of dead skin cells, revealing the younger skin underneath.

It is simple to use. Just place it on a washcloth and gently work it into a rich, creamy lather as you cleanse your skin with it, and then thoroughly rinse off. Do not use it for your face, though, as it's too aggressive and is meant for the body only. This one is quite inexpensive, costing as little as $3.50 for a large bottle.

OTHER BEAUTY ISSUES

Thinning Hair

One of the newest treatments for thinning hair is **platelet-rich plasma (PRP)**. I mentioned PRP earlier with microneedling. To make PRP, a sample of blood is taken from a person's arm, and then the blood's platelets and plasma are separated from the red blood cells. This PRP is full of growth factors. It is then injected into areas of the scalp with thinning hair, encouraging the hair to enter an active growth phase. This can cause the hair to thicken.

Early anecdotal reports reveal that three to four months are needed to see results, and the treatments must be repeated at least once a year to maintain the hair's thickness. Since there are currently so many noninvasive options for thinning hair (like Rogaine, low-light lasers, and dietary changes), PRP isn't my first choice of treatment. However, it is an exciting new option that warrants further investigation.

As an aside, PRP has been used for the past several years in a lot of other treatments. Orthopedic surgeons have used it to help speed healing, plastic surgeons have used it to decrease bleeding with facelifts, and dermatologists have used it with microneedling. The science supporting all these applications is still limited, but many doctors believe in the magic of PRP.

Tattoo Regret

It seems that everyone under the age of thirty-five has at least one tattoo, usually more. Experts are projecting that the number of individuals seeking to get rid of their tattoos will dramatically rise over the next five to ten years. So, what's the best way to get rid of unwanted ink?

In the past, we had to use a separate laser to destroy each individual color in the tattoo. Red ink would require one laser, blue ink another laser, and so on. These nanosecond lasers would often require up to ten treatments and achieve only a 60 percent clearance rate, sometimes leaving ghostly hues of colors behind. Not a good look.

Enter the newest lasers: the picosecond lasers. These devices fire much more quickly (in mere picoseconds), causing them to be significantly more effective in blasting away tattoo ink. Three devices are currently available: **PicoSure** (the original), **PicoWay**, and **Enlighten**. All three appear to be far superior in clearing tattoos to the older, nanosecond lasers. They are more effective and require fewer treatments. So, if you regret your tattoos, try to see a doctor who has one of these picosecond lasers.

Dry Skin of the Hands

In chapter 9, I give a number of solutions for dry, cracked skin of the hands. Most of them require several steps, but here's an easy, effective way to rejuvenate and rehydrate your hands without doing anything but wearing a pair of gloves. **Borghese Spa Mani Moisture Restoring Gloves** are infused with hydrating emollients (olive oil, grape-seed oil, ceramides, and vitamin E) that restore moisture to dry, cracked hands. You can wear them for a twenty-minute mini session or an overnight intense rehydrating treatment. Although they're somewhat costly at $49, these gloves can be reused for up to three months. Just put them on your hands in the evening while you're watching TV, and very quickly your hands will be soft and silky.

SUPERFOOD SWITCHES TO LOOK YEARS YOUNGER

As you read in chapter 5, the food we eat can have profound effects on how our skin looks and how quickly we age. Therefore, any antiaging plan should include a healthy, Age

Fix–approved diet. Sometimes, the easiest ways to change our diet and eat healthier is to make small switches. For instance, if you're a die-hard soda pop fan, then to stop drinking it all of a sudden and exchange it for ice water could be a real challenge. So, be realistic when changing your diet to eat more nutritious and skin-friendly foods. Make small changes each week or month, and these changes will build up over time. Here are some easy but effective food switches to consider:

1. **Switch Coffee to Green Tea**

   Green tea might be the most powerful of all the antioxidant sources. The polyphenols in green tea have been shown to be one hundred times more effective than vitamin C in fighting free radicals. Now, many people who drink coffee consume several cups per day. This might be you. If that's the case, then making the cold-turkey switch from coffee to green tea could be pretty difficult.

   Here's a solution: Start slowly. If you drink three cups of coffee per day, begin by decreasing to two cups of coffee and adding one cup of green tea. After a few weeks, go down to one cup of coffee and go up to two cups of green tea. A few weeks later, discontinue the coffee altogether for green tea. You'll still get your much-desired caffeine boost but with more antioxidants and fewer unhealthy additives (sugar, cream, etc.).

2. **Switch Cream Cheese to Almond Butter on Your Bagel**

   My kids love to slather cream cheese on their bagels. Unfortunately, cream cheese isn't all that healthy and doesn't make your skin any younger. So, try substituting almond butter for cream cheese. Not only is almond butter tasty, it's also full of healthy monounsaturated fatty acids. Unlike saturated and trans fats, which are inflammatory and accelerate the aging process, monounsaturated fatty acids are anti-inflammatory. They soothe and calm the skin, protect it from UV radiation, and even moisturize the skin from the inside out.

   Some of my friends and patients complain that almond butter tastes too dry. If this applies to you, then try a natural peanut butter. Make sure to avoid peanut butter with too many additives and preservatives, and avoid low-fat peanut butter, which often has an extra dose of unhealthy sugar to take the place of the missing healthy peanut fat.

3. **Switch Milk Chocolate to Dark Chocolate**

   Raw cocoa contains an enormous dose of free-radical-fighting antioxidants. Chocolate bars are graded according to how much raw cocoa (or cacao, same thing) they contain. The higher the percentage of raw cocoa, the higher the antioxidant content. Unfortunately, most commercially available chocolate bars, like milk chocolate or even Hershey's Dark, contain too much sugar and too little cocoa to be healthy for you. So, if you like chocolate—and who doesn't?—then try to stick with or switch to dark chocolate with at least 70 percent raw cocoa.

This also pertains to hot chocolate. Instant hot chocolate usually contains too much sugar and too many additives—and too little cocoa—to give a beneficial effect. Instead, try making your own dark hot chocolate at home. Just mix organic, unsweetened ground cocoa with almond milk and a touch of honey or stevia. Yum!

4. **Switch Vegetable Oil to Avocado Oil**

Which oil is the best for you? It can be very confusing. Back in the 1980s, everyone thought margarine was much healthier than butter. We now know that margarine contains trans fats (called partially hydrogenated vegetable oil on packaging) and that these trans fats are not safe. Vegetable oil can also contain too much omega-6 fatty acid, which can be inflammatory to our bodies.

Currently, it appears that avocado oil, even more than olive oil, may be the best oil for preventing and slowing down the aging process. Although avocado oil contains a similar amount of monounsaturated fatty acids as olive oil, it contains fewer harmful saturated fats and more of the healthy omega-3 fatty acids than olive oil. It also has a very high smoking point, making it ideal for both low-temperature uses (e.g., drizzling it on a salad) and extremely high-temperature uses (e.g., pan-searing meats). It's also full of carotenoid antioxidants and can even increase the absorption of carotenoids from other foods. I encourage you to try avocado oil if you haven't.

5. **Switch Croutons to Sunflower Seeds**

Croutons are basically empty calories. They are usually made with refined white bread and may also contain additives, such as salt. Instead of croutons, try sprinkling some sunflower seeds on your salad. Sunflower seeds are great sources of vitamin E, vitamin B, and copper.

I hope you've enjoyed reading this extra chapter and have found some new and exciting ways to turn back the clock. Throughout *The Age Fix* I've recommended skin-care products of all different types, costs, and manufacturers. Although these products have passed my most important test—they work—some of them contain ingredients that aren't natural and may even be controversial. To those of you who are interested in natural, organic skin-care products, I want you to know that I hear you. By the time you are reading this, I will have launched my very own skin-care line: YOUN Beauty. It's a complete line of anti-aging skin-care products that are natural, organic, not tested on animals, and free of sulfates, parabens, dyes, and phthalates. Not only are they safe to use, but they work. YOUN Beauty products can be purchased online for your convenience.

If you like what you've read in this book, please follow me on Facebook and visit my website at www.dryoun.com to sign up for my free e-newsletter. Every couple of weeks I'll email you the latest tips, tricks, and secrets to looking and feeling younger.

Please join me. I'd love to meet you.

Let's look, live, and be better.

Sincerely,

Anthony Youn, MD

America's Holistic Plastic Surgeon

ACKNOWLEDGMENTS

First, and always first, thanks be to God, for blessing me beyond my wildest dreams. Great is thy faithfulness to me.

To my beautiful and wonderful wife, Amy. Thank you for always being supportive of my many endeavors. You are my treasure, and I am so thankful to have you in my life.

To Mom and Dad. Thank you for always being proud of me. I love you.

To Eve Adamson. I couldn't have asked for a better collaborator. You were an absolute joy to work with. Thank you for creating *The Age Fix* with me.

To Wendy Sherman, my agent extraordinaire. You will always have my eternal gratitude for your encouragement and belief in this project. I couldn't do this without you!

To my editor, Sarah Pelz. You are a lovely person, inside and out. Thank you for all your interest and for bringing me under your wing. I am so incredibly blessed to work with you.

To the team at Grand Central Life and Style, especially Jamie Raab and Karen Murgolo. Thank you for making me a part of your family. I am indebted to each one of you and proud to be one of your authors.

To Matt Cushman, the artist behind the *Age Fix* illustrations. Who would've thought that we'd end up working on this more than thirty years after meeting in Greenville? Mike Hillary would be proud. Thanks for all your hard work.

To dermatologist Dr. Emily Levin. Thank you for taking the time to review my chapters on skin care. I look forward to reading Peter's next book!

To celebrity nutritionist Maria Bella. Thank you for your helpful suggestions on the Age-Fix diet.

To my aestheticians Chris Krebs and Paula Scott. Thank you for all your help with this project, including suggesting products and reviewing my makeup tips, and especially for being my guinea pigs.

To Rachael Ray and everyone at the *Rachael Ray* show. Thank you for always supporting me and making me look good. It's an honor to work with all of you.

To Dr. Mike Dow. Thank you for suggesting that I write a book on looking younger. See you in the next greenroom!

To Dr. Brian Smith. Our writing journey continues! It means a lot to me that we're in this together.

To Jim and Py, Lisa and Mike (and Toki, too). Thank you for being my closest family and biggest cheerleaders.

To all my friends and family who have been so supportive, interested, and involved with my writing. My relationships with you mean everything to me. There are too many of you to list, but please be aware that I really appreciate your love, support, and ribbing through the years. Thank you, thank you, thank you!

To my employees: Renee, X-tina, Jenny, Megan, Dev, Andrea, and Kelly. Thank you for being my support staff, dealing with my crazy schedule, and taking such good care of me and my patients. Don't leave!

To Dr. Danielle DeLuca-Pytell. Thank you for covering for me when I'm out (and making sure no one sleeps on my couch!).

To my patients, past and present. I cannot put in words how much I appreciate your trust in me. I couldn't be what I am, and do what I do, without you. It's a privilege to be your doctor.

To everyone who purchased *The Age Fix* and *In Stitches*. Thank you for spending your hard-earned money to read my writing. I truly appreciate it, especially your nice messages, letters, and reviews. They make the hundreds of hours I spend typing on my computer worthwhile. See you on Twitter (@tonyyounmd), Instagram, and Facebook!

And finally, to D and G. Your daddy is always so proud of you. I love you two more than anything.

APPENDIX 1

Product Sources

I mention many products, tools, and gadgets in this book, and you probably want more information on where you can buy the things that interest you the most. To help you out, I've listed everything I've mentioned that you may want to buy. For each entry, I'll let you know whether it is available over the counter, in a physician's office, or by prescription only. I'll also let you know the suggested retail price (you can often find things cheaper on sale or online). Keep in mind that prices may change, so the prices given here are current estimates. To make it easiest for you, visit my website, **www.dryoun.com**, for links to purchase most of these products online. Happy shopping!

Key:

OTC = Over the Counter

PO = Physician's Office

RX = Prescription Required

$ = Under $10

$$ = $10–$25

$$$ = $26–$50

$$$$ = $50+

CHAPTER 2:

Juverest Sleep Wrinkle Pillow, $$$$, OTC,
www.juverest.com, $179.00. An extra cover costs $39.50.

UV protection clothing:

* Solumbra, sunprecautions.com

* Coolibar, coolibar.com

* Solartex, solartex.com

CHAPTER 3:

Alpha-Hydroxy Acid (AHA), $$, OTC, as low as $15 at your local drugstore

Bioré Deep Cleansing Pore Strips, $, OTC, www.biore.com, 14 nose strips for under $10

Dermablend concealer, $$$, OTC, www.dermablend.com

Frownies, $$, OTC, www.frownies.com, $19.95 per box

L'Oréal RevitaLift, $$, OTC, www.lorealparisusa.com, $17.99 per jar

L'Oréal Youth Code skin-care line, $$$, OTC, www.lorealparisusa.com

La Roche-Posay Thermal Spring Water, $$, OTC, www.laroche-posay.us, $12.99

Obagi Nu-Derm, $$$$, PO, www.obagi.com, sold exclusively through physicians

Peter Thomas Roth's Un-Wrinkle Peel Pads, $$$, OTC, www.peterthomasroth.com, $45 for 60 pads

Retin-A (tretinoin), an **AGE FIX FAVORITE**, $$$, RX, $40–$50 at local pharmacy with online coupon—just Google it to find it (otherwise over $75 per tube)

Silk'n FaceFX, $$$$, OTC, www.silkn.com/facefx, special offer of $149 plus a free jar of the Dead Sea Mineral Cream and free shipping

Tanda Zap, $$$, OTC, www.tanda.com, $39.99

Teoxane Cosmeceuticals, an **AGE FIX FAVORITE**, $$$$, PO, www.teoxane.com (Full disclosure: I am a shareholder in Alphaeon, the company that dispenses Teoxane in the United States.)

ZO Medical skin-care line, $$$$, PO, shop.zoskinhealth.com, sold exclusively through physicians

CHAPTER 4:

Avène Extremely Gentle Cleansing Lotion, $$$, OTC, www.aveneusa.com, $20 online at Amazon.com

Avène Thermal Spring Water spray, $, OTC, www.aveneusa.com, $16 on Amazon.com

CE Ferulic, an ✱ AGE FIX FAVORITE, $$$$, OTC, www.skinceuticals.com, $157

CeraVe Hydrating Cleanser $, OTC, www.cerave.com, $10 at Target

Clarisonic, $$$$, OTC, www.clarisonic.com, devices start at $100

Clinique Rinse-Off Foaming Cleanser, $$, OTC, www.clinique.com, $20

Effaclar Pore Refining Anti-Wrinkle Serum, $$$, OTC, www.laroche-posay.us, $44.99 for a 30 ml bottle

Epicuren Micro-Derm Ultra-Refining Scrub, $$$, OTC, www.epicuren.com, $27 for a 0.5 oz. tube

Epionce Gentle Foaming Cleanser, $$$, OTC, www.epionce.com, $32

L'Oréal Youth Code (see chapter 3)

La Roche-Posay Anthelios, $$$, OTC, www.laroche-posay.us/anthelios, 5 fl. oz. for $35.99

NARS Multi-Action Hydrating Toner, $$$, OTC, www.narscosmetics.com, $32

Neocutis Bio-Restorative Serum, $$$$, PO, www.neocutis.com, $235 on dermstore.com

NEOVA Crème de la Copper, $$$$, OTC, www.neova.com, $110 for 1.7 fl. oz.

NEOVA Progressive Nourishing Lotion, $$$$, OTC, www.neova.com, $95 for 1.7 fl. oz.

Neutrogena Fresh Foaming Cleaner, $, OTC, www.neutrogena.com, $4.99 at Target

Neutrogena Rapid Wrinkle Repair, $$, OTC, www.neutrogena.com, $20.99

Neutrogena Wave, $$, OTC, www.neutrogena.com, $16.99 for the spinning power cleanser

Oil of Olay Regenerist line, $$, OTC, www.olay.com, prices range from $8.99 to $25.99

Olay's Professional Pro-X Advanced Cleansing System, $$$, OTC, www.olay.com, $29.99 for the brush and the exfoliating cleanser

Olay Regenerist Night Recovery Cream, $$, OTC, www.olay.com, $22.99

Philosophy Purity Made Simple Cleanser, $, OTC, www.philosophy.com, $10 for a 3 oz. bottle

Pond's Cold Cream Cleanser, $, OTC, www.ponds.com, around $5 at your local drugstore

ReFissa, $$$$, PO, www.refissa.com, around $75

Renova, $$$$, PO, RX, prescription only, around $75

Revision Retinol Facial Repair, $$$, PO, www.revisionskincare.com, around $55, sold at physician's office

RoC Retinol Correxion cream, $$, OTC, www.rocskincare.com, $22.99

SkinCeuticals Retinol 1.0, $$$$, OTC, www.skinceuticals.com, $63

SkinMedica's TNS Essential Serum, $$$$, OTC, www.skinmedica.com, $270

StriVectin's Advanced Intensive Concentrate for Wrinkles and Stretch Marks, $$$$, OTC, www.strivectin.com, $139 for a 4.5 oz. bottle

Teoxane RHA Serum, an ✳ AGE FIX FAVORITE , $$$$, PO, www.alphaeon.com/products, $190

TNS Recovery Complex, $$$$, OTC, www.skinmedica.com, $172

ZO Medical C-Bright, $$$$, PO, shop.zoskinhealth.com, $90

ZO Medical Cebatrol Oil Control Pads, $$$$, PO, www.shopzoskinhealth.com, $62

ZO Multi-Therapy Hydroquinone System, an ✳ AGE FIX FAVORITE , $$$$, PO, shop.zoskinhealth.com, available through physician's office

ZO Skin Health's Offects Exfoliating Polish, $$$$, OTC, shop.zoskinhealth.com, $65

ZO Skin Health's Ommerse Overnight Recovery Crème, $$$$, OTC, shop .zoskinhealth.com, $100 for 1.7 fl. oz.

CHAPTER 6:

Art Harding's Instant Facelift, $$$, OTC, www.instantfacelifts.com, $25 for a 22-piece kit

Athena 7 Minute Lift, $$$$, OTC, www.7minutelift.com, 1 jar is a 60-day supply for $79

Breast and Chest Pillow from Intimia, $$$, OTC, www.intimia.com, $49.95

Burt's Bees lip balm, $, OTC, www.burtsbees.com, 4-pack of lip balms for $10

Epicuren Instantlift Facial Cream, $$$$, OTC, www.epicuren.com, $108

Facelift Bungee, $$, OTC, www.faceliftbungee.com, $24.99

L'Oréal's Revitalift Miracle Blur, $$, OTC, www.lorealparisusa.com, $24.99

Lobe Wonder, $, OTC, www.lobewonder.com, 60 patches per box for $6

Lytera Skin Brightening Complex, $$$$, OTC, www.skinmedica.com, $125 and free shipping

Pillow Bra, $$$$, OTC, www.pillowbra.com, €57, roughly $72

Sexy Mother Pucker Lip Plumping Gloss, $$, OTC, www.sephora.com, $18

CHAPTER 7:

DERMAdoctor Wrinkle Revenge Rescue and Protect Eye Balm, $$$, OTC, www .dermadoctor.com, $50

Dr. Brandt Revitalizing Retinol Eye Cream, $$$$, OTC, www.drbrandtskincare .com, $55

Elastilash, $$$$, OTC, www.obagi.com, $74.98 on Amazon.com

Instant Forehead Smoother, $$$$, OTC, www.bremennclinical.com, $69

Latisse, an ✱ AGE FIX FAVORITE, $$$$, PO, www.latisse.com, sold exclusively through physicians

Marini Lash, $$$$, OTC, www.janmarini.com, $60 for a 2-month supply

Murad Time Release Retinol Concentrate, $$$$, OTC, www.murad.com, $65

Nutra-Lift Instant Results Anti-Aging Firming Cream, $$$$, OTC, www.nutra-lift .com, 2 oz. jar for $62

Olay Regenerist Luminous Dark Circle Correcting Hydraswirl, $$$, OTC, www .olay.com, $25.99

Revision D·E·J Eye Cream, $$$$, PO, www.revisionskincare.com, sold exclusively through physicians, $85

Revision Retinol Eye Repair, $$$$, PO, www.revisionskincare.com, sold exclusively through physicians, approximately $70

Revitalash, $$$$, OTC, www.revitalash.com, $98 for a 3-month supply

RoC Retinol Correxion eye cream, $$, OTC, www.rocskincare.com, $22.99

Sudden Change Under-Eye Firming Serum, an 🌸 **AGE FIX FAVORITE**, $$, OTC, www.suddenchange.com, 2-pack for $19.99

ZO Medical Hydrafirm, an 🌸 **AGE FIX FAVORITE**, $$$$, PO, shop.zoskinhealth.com, $140

CHAPTER 8:

Adonia LegTone Serum, an 🌸 **AGE FIX FAVORITE**, $$$$, OTC, www.legtone.com, $79 per bottle (a 60-day supply)

Adonia Tummy Tone, $$$$, OTC, www.tummytone.com, $79 per bottle (a 60-day supply)

Bubbles Bodywear, $$$, OTC, www.lovemybubbles.com, $46 for the "Double O" butt lifter

Dr. Rey Shapewear, $$$, OTC, www.classicshapewear.com, ranges from $25 to $55 per garment

Fat Girl Slim, $$$, OTC, www.sephora.com, $36 for a 6-oz. jar

Kojilac CHQ Pads, an 🌸 **AGE FIX FAVORITE**, $$$$, PO, Approximately $80, sold exclusively through physicians

Suddenly Slender, $$$$, OTC, www.suddenlyslender.com, $289 for the at-home package

Wellbox, $$$$, OTC, www.wellbox.com, $1,499 for the machine

CHAPTER 9:

BioCorneum, $$$$, PO, www.biocorneum.com, around $70 for a 20-gram bottle, sold exclusively through physicians

Burt's Bees Almond Milk Beeswax Hand Crème, $, OTC, www.burtsbees.com, $8.99 at Target

Crest 3D White toothpaste, an **AGE FIX FAVORITE**, $, OTC, www.3dwhite.com, $5.99 at Target

Eucerin Intensive Repair Extra-Enriched Hand Cream, $, OTC, www.eucerinus.com, $5.49 at Walgreens

Heel Rescue Superior Moisturizing Foot Cream, $$, OTC, available for purchase at Amazon.com

Neutrogena Norwegian Formula Hand Cream, an **AGE FIX FAVORITE**, $, OTC, www.neutrogena.com, $4.79 at Walgreens

ProFresh, $$$, OTC, www.profresh.com, $39.99 for the starter kit

Propecia, $$$$, PO, prescription required

Rogaine, $$$, OTC, www.rogaine.com, $29.99 for a 2-month supply

Silagen, $$$$, PO, www.silagen.com, $70 for a 30-gram pump bottle, sold exclusively through physicians

Silk'n Flash&Go, an **AGE FIX FAVORITE**, $$$$, OTC, www.silkn.com, $199

Silk'n Pedi, an **AGE FIX FAVORITE**, $$$, OTC, www.silkn.com, $29 at Target

Therafirm tights, $$$$, OTC, www.therafirm.com, range from $37.95 to $84.95

Tria Hair Removal Laser 4X, $$$$, OTC, www.triabeauty.com, $475 for the deluxe kit

APPENDIX 2

If You Need a Plastic Surgeon

You may never need a plastic surgeon, but if you do, then I implore you: Do your homework so that you work only with someone who is experienced, reputable, ethical, and fully qualified.

The way to do this is, first of all, to find a plastic surgeon who is certified by the **American Board of Plastic Surgery (ABPS)**, the only plastic surgery board that is recognized by the American Board of Medical Specialties (ABMS), and a member of the **American Society of Plastic Surgeons (ASPS)**. Nearly all board-certified plastic surgeons are members of ASPS, including surgeons who specialize in reconstructive surgery. If you are more interested in cosmetic procedures, look for plastic surgeons who are members of the **American Society for Aesthetic Plastic Surgery (ASAPS)**. The top board-certified plastic surgeons who specialize in cosmetic surgery are members of ASAPS and represent the pinnacle of cosmetic plastic surgeons.

There are also some subspecialty qualifications to look for:

* **For facial plastic surgery:** Look for a doctor certified by the **American Board of Facial Plastic and Reconstructive Surgery (ABFPRS)**. This certification is considered equivalent to certification by the American Board of Plastic Surgery in all states, so choosing a member of ABFPRS is reasonable for plastic surgery of the face. Unfortunately, some facial plastic surgeons are delving into plastic surgery of the body (such as breast implants). I've seen many nightmare cases of botched breast implant surgery by facial plastic surgeons, so reserve facial plastic surgeons for procedures of the face!

* **For cosmetic eyelid surgery:** Look for members of the **American Society for Ophthalmic Plastic and Reconstructive Surgery**. They are well trained to perform plastic surgery of the eyelids (as are surgeons certified by the ABPS and ABFPRS).

* **For anything else:** Remember this—surgeons certified by the **American Board of Plastic Surgery** are trained for plastic surgery of the entire face and body. When in doubt, choose one of these.

There are many other "boards" and "societies" out there. In fact, I could legally make my own "Dr. Youn's Board of Age Fix Surgery" and certify doctors with it if I wanted to do that (which, thankfully, I do not). The ones I've mentioned above are the only ones that I give my stamp of approval to.

There are some other ways to vet your surgeon, however.

* **Let your hospital do the work.** One good way is to use the resources of your hospital. Hospitals will vet surgeons before hiring them, and typically allow surgeons to perform only operations that they are qualified to perform. Therefore, make sure your doctor has privileges to perform the surgery you want at a hospital. Phony plastic surgeons get around this by performing their operations in their own in-office operating rooms, but they are not allowed in hospitals.

* **Check online for doctor-rating websites.** There are multiple online doctor-rating websites where patients can rate their doctors and write about their experiences with their physicians. For plastic surgery, the best one is currently **RealSelf.com**. Use these, but also take these reviews with a grain of salt. There are reports of patients spamming these sites, posting multiple negative (or positive) experiences about the same doctor as a way to punish them for what they perceive as (but which might not necessarily have been) poor care. There are also reports of doctors writing bad reviews for their competitors! Unethical, but it happens.

* **Check your state's board of medicine website.** You want to make sure your doctor's medical license hasn't been put on probation, suspended, or, even worse, revoked.

* **Check your county courts.** In most cases, malpractice cases are considered public information, and some county courts allow you to look these up online. Keep in mind, though, that we live in a very litigious society. Even the best surgeons get sued, often more than once. However, if your doctor has a long list of malpractice lawsuits, then you may want to take this into account. You can also check to see if your doctor has been in the courts for something more serious, like drug-related offenses. I know of several surgeons who have gotten in hot water for prescription drug abuse. Drug abusers are not necessarily the type of doctors you want cutting you open.

✳ **Ask your local nurses or other hospital employees.** These employees talk, and they typically have a good sense of who the good and bad doctors are. If you're really connected, talk with someone who works in the OR, either a surgical nurse, nurse anesthetist, or scrub technician, as they are the ones who actually see the plastic surgeons operate. They know who has steady hands, who's meticulous, who rushes through the surgery, and who has the most complications. They might not be willing to dish on the details of who to avoid, but if you are lucky, they might at least give you a thumbs-up or a concerned frown.

✳ **Ask your family doctor.** Not all family doctors are knowledgeable about who the good plastic surgeons are, but it's one more opinion that may turn out to be valuable.

NOTES

1   Photoprotection by window glass, automobile glass, and sunglasses. Tuchinda C, Srivannaboon S, Lim HW. *Journal of the American Academy of Dermatology*, May 2006; 54(5):845–54.

2   Ambient solar UVR, personal exposure and protection. Gies P, et al. *Journal of Epidemiology*, 1999; 9:S115–S122.

3   Fat redistribution following suction lipectomy: defense of body fat and patterns of restoration. Hernandez TL, et al. *Obesity* (Silver Spring), July 2011; 19(7):1388–95.

4   Prospective study of lidocaine, bupivacaine, and epinephrine levels and blood loss in patients undergoing liposuction and abdominoplasty. Swanson E. *Plastic and Reconstructive Surgery*, September 2012; 130(3):702–22.

5   The relationship between basal and squamous cell skin cancer and smoking related cancers. Sitas F, et al. *BMC Research Notes,* 2011; 4:556; http://www.biomedcentral.com/1756-0500/4/556.
    Also see: Relation between smoking and skin cancer. De Hertog SAE, et al. *Journal of Clinical Oncology,* January 1, 2001; 19(1):231–38.

6   Cigarette smoking associated with premature facial wrinkling: image analysis of facial skin replicas. Jae Sook Koh, et al. *International Journal of Dermatology*, January 2002; 41(1):21–27.

7   Cigarette smoking: risk factor for premature facial wrinkling. Kadunce DP, et al. *Annals of Internal Medicine*, May 15, 1991; 114(10):840–44.

8   Multicenter randomized comparative double-blind controlled clinical trial of the safety and efficacy of zinc gluconate versus minocycline hydrochloride in the treatment of inflammatory acne vulgaris. Dreno B, et al. *Dermatology*, 2001; 203(2):135–40.

9   Effect of zinc gluconate on propionibacterium acnes resistance to erythromycin in patients with inflammatory acne: in vitro and in vivo study. Dreno B, et al. *European Journal of Dermatology*, January 2005; 15(3):152–55.

10 Statistics and facts on the cosmetic industry. The Statistics Portal. http://www.statista.com/topics/1008/cosmetics-industry/.

11 Do plastic micro-beads from facial scrubbers escape sewage treatment? Wilson, S. *Our Blog*, April 16, 2013. 5Gyres Institute. http://5gyres.org/posts/2013/04/16/do_plastic_micro_beads_from_facial_scrubbers_escape_sewage_treatment/.

12 Retinoids for prevention and treatment of actinic keratosis. Ianhez M, et al. *Anais Brasileiros de Dermatologia*, July–August 2013; 88(4):585–93. http://www.ncbi.nlm.nih.gov/pmc/articles/PMC3760934/.

13 UV photoprotection by combination topical antioxidants vitamin C and vitamin E. Lin JY, et al. *Journal of the American Academy of Dermatology*, June 2003; 48(6):866–74.

14 Collagen stimulating effect of peptide amphiphile C16-KTTKS on human fibroblasts. Jones RR, et al. *Molecular Pharmaceutics*, March 2013; 10(3):1063–69.

15 GABA$_A$ receptors are expressed and facilitate relaxation in airway smooth muscle. Mizuta K, et al. *American Journal of Physiology—Lung Cellular and Molecular Physiology*, June 1, 2008; 294(6):L1206–L1216.

16 Factors contributing to the facial aging of identical twins. Guyuron B, et al. *Plastic and Reconstructive Surgery*, 2009; 123(4):1321–31.

17 Nutrition and acne. Danby FW. *Clinics in Dermatology*, November–December 2010; 28(6):598–604.

18 Soda and cell aging: associations between sugar-sweetened beverage consumption and leukocyte telomere length in healthy adults from the National Health and Nutrition Examination Surveys. Leung CW, et al. *American Journal of Public Health*, December 2014; 104(12):2425–31. http://ajph.aphapublications.org/doi/abs/10.2105/AJPH.2014.302151?journalCode=ajph&; and also here: http://www.washingtonpost.com/news/morning-mix/wp/2014/10/20/sugary-sodas-could-take-4-6-years-off-your-life/.

19 At the time of this book's printing, this list was located here: http://www.health.harvard.edu/newsweek/Glycemic_index_and_glycemic_load_for_100_foods.htm.

20 Factors contributing to the facial aging of identical twins. Guyuron, B, et al. *Plastic and Reconstructive Surgery*, 2009; 123(4):1321–31.

21 Skin wrinkling: can food make a difference? Purba MB, et al. *Journal of the American College of Nutrition*, February 2001; 20(1):71–80.

22 Dietary nutrient intakes and skin-aging appearance among middle-aged American women. Cogrove M, et al. *American Journal of Clinical Nutrition*, October 2007; 86(4):1225–31.

23 Antioxidant activity of blueberry fruit is impaired by association with milk. Serafini M, et al. *Free Radical Biology and Medicine*, March 15, 2009; 46(6):769–74.

24 Tomatoes "help keep skin young" and protect against sunburn. Hope J. *Daily Mail* (UK), June 6, 2012. http://www.dailymail.co.uk/health/article-2155595/Tomatoes-help-skin-young-protect-sunburn.html.

25 Jenkins G, et al. *International Journal of Cosmetic Science*, February 2014; 36(1):22–31.

26 Fruits and vegetables that are sources for lutein and zeaxanthin: the macular pigment in human eyes. Sommerburg O, et al. *British Journal of Ophthalmology*, August 1998; 82(8):907–10.

27 Drink green tea for your good health. September 12, 1997. University of Kansas. Office of Public Affairs. http://www.oread.ku.edu/Oread97/OreadSept12/page1/tea.html.

28 Dietary nutrient intakes and skin-aging appearance among middle-aged American women. Cogrove M, et al. *American Journal of Clinical Nutrition*, October 2007; 86(4):1225–31.

29 Better psychological functioning and higher social status may largely explain the apparent health benefits of wine: a study of wine and beer drinking in young Danish adults. Mortensen EL, et al. *Archives of Internal Medicine*, August 13–27, 2011; 161(15):1844–48.

30 The SMAS and the nasolabial fold. Barton, FE, Jr. *Plastic and Reconstructive Surgery*, June 1992; 89(6):1054–57.

31 The effect of acute exercise on serum brain-derived neurotrophic factor levels and cognitive function. Ferris LT, Williams JS, and Shen CL. *Medicine and Science in Sports and Exercise*, April 2007; 39(4):728–34. Beneficial effects of long-term endurance exercise on leukocyte telomere biology. Werner C, et al. *Circulation*, 2009; 120:S492. Low-intensity daily walking activity is associated with hippocampal volume in older adults. Varma VR, et al. *Hippocampus*, December 7, 2014; doi: 10.1002/hipo.22397.

32   Exercise as a countermeasure for aging: from mice to humans. Tarnopolsky, M. Presented at the twenty-third annual meeting of the American Medical Society for Sports Medicine, April 16, 2014.

33   Radiofrequency and 585-nm pulsed dye laser treatment of striae distensae: a report of 37 Asian patients. Suh DH, et al. *Dermatologic Surgery*, January 2007; 33(1):29–34.

34   Comparison of efficacy of silicone gel, silicone gel sheeting, and topical onion extract including heparin and allantoin for the treatment of postburn hypertrophic scars. Karagoz H, et al. *Journal of the International Society for Burn Injuries*, December 2009; 35(8):1097–103.

35   Adjuvant single-fraction radiotherapy is safe and effective for intractable keloids. Song C, et al. *Journal of Radiation Research*, September 2014; 55(5):912–16.

36   Microneedling for acne scars in Asian skin type: an effective low cost treatment modality. Dogra S, Yadav S, and Sarangal R. *Journal of Cosmetic Dermatology*, September 2014; 13(3):180–87.

37   Average reduction in fat volume following single treatment as measured by MRI; "Clinical and Histological Evaluations of a 1060nm Laser Device for Non-Invasive Fat Reduction." John W. Decorato, MD, FACS; Rafael Sierra, PhD; and Bo Chen, PhD. Westford, MA, 2014.

INDEX

ABOUT DR. ANTHONY YOUN

Anthony Youn, MD, is a nationally recognized, board-certified plastic surgeon who is considered one of the country's best-known experts in looking younger with or without surgery. Recognized as a leader in his field, Dr. Youn is valued for his honest approach and ability to speak to all areas of health and well-being.

More than being a regular expert on the *Rachael Ray* show, *The Dr. Oz Show*, and *The Doctors*, Dr. Youn's expertise has also been featured on *Good Morning America*, *Katie*, *Today*, *CBS This Morning*, *Access Hollywood*, Fox News, CNN, HLN, *E!*, *HuffPost Live*, and in the *New York Times*, *USA Today*, *People* magazine, *InTouch*, *Life and Style*, and *Us Weekly*, just to name a few. Dr. Youn is also a regular contributor for CNN.com, NBCNews.com, and the *Huffington Post*.

A national lecturer, Dr. Youn has published several scientific articles in peer-reviewed journals, and he has also published *In Stitches*, his critically acclaimed and award-winning memoir of becoming a doctor (Gallery Books/Simon and Schuster, 2011). Named a "Top Plastic Surgeon" by *U.S. News and World Report* and *Harper's Bazaar*, Dr. Youn serves on the Editorial Advisory Board for *Plastic Surgery Practice Magazine* and is a member of the American Society of Plastic Surgeons (ASPS), American Society for Aesthetic Plastic Surgery (ASAPS), and a fellow of the American College of Surgeons. He is an assistant professor of surgery at the Oakland University William Beaumont School of Medicine.

For more information, please visit: www.dryoun.com.